Commendations ... all

"In the journey of life it is a rare thing to find a true and loyal friend. I first met Adrian Adger in 1991 and I regard him as my best friend. It was heartbreaking when Adrian was diagnosed with cancer but, with God's help, he has stood tall and he has recaptured the joy of the Lord. It is an honour to endorse my best friend, and the reading of his life's story."

Rev Brian Smyth, *Trinity Presbyterian Church, Ahoghill*

"If you come from Belfast you are one of two things, 'Big' or 'Wee'. Everyone knows a big Albert or a wee Albert, everyone knows a big Aggie or a wee Aggie – that's just the way it is. When Adrian Adger joined the ranks of the Belfast City Mission in 1994, his colleagues quickly gave him the title 'Big Adrian' – obviously because of his stature (over six and a half feet tall). We on the staff were soon to find out that he also was big in heart, big into the Word of God, big into sharing that Word through his passionate preaching, big into fervent prayer, big into mission and big into soul-winning for his Saviour. I heartily endorse this book of Adrian's that will reveal his genuineness and deep faith in the Lord Jesus Christ, even in the midst of adversity."

Bobi Brown, *Executive Secretary, Belfast City Mission*

"With courageous and vivid honesty, Adrian answers many challenging questions that people, including Christians, often confront when they discover they have incurable cancer. This book presents hope and encouragement as we read how Adrian's vibrant relationship with God, alongside his desire and commitment to share his faith and put his trust in God, enables him to live with joy as he navigates life with incurable cancer."

Dr Cherith Semple, *Cancer Care Specialist*

"This is an inspiring story presented with humour, honesty and deep humility. Since being gripped by divine grace, Adrian has been grounded in the Scriptures and guided by the Holy Spirit.

Thus when he received a devastating medical diagnosis and faced unexpected suffering, he was enabled to address the difficult and challenging questions with a resolute confidence in the faithfulness of a Sovereign Lord who had repeatedly proven true to His Word over earlier years. This book is a vibrant testimony to the stabilising reality of the promises of God in the face of earth's uncertainties and unanswerable questions. I recommend it warmly to a wide readership."

Rev Dr John Dixon, *former moderator of Presbyterian Church in Ireland*

"Adrian has faced his battle with cancer with tremendous fortitude. Resting on the promises of God, realising the presence of God, relying on the providence of God he has continued to faithfully preach the Word and carry out his pastoral responsibilities. He has proved God's grace in a wonderful way. I commend this book to you and trust that God be glorified through this production."

Denis Lyle, *Baptist pastor*

"It is my immense privilege to heartily commend this book. I have treasured my friendship with Adrian for these past years and hold him in the highest possible esteem as an outstanding servant of Christ. He has blessed me through his friendship and ministry, just as he has blessed Mission Africa, the Church in Nigeria and, of course, the church in Northern Ireland. It is a further blessing to see his Christian journey and reflections set down for us in these pages. I am struck afresh by his spiritual vitality, his humility before the Lord and his deep prayerfulness. Adrian—both in person and on the written page – is an inspiration as he points us to the Saviour that he serves and proclaims."

Rev Dr Paul Bailie, *CEO of Mission Africa*

Facing Cancer Standing Tall

One Christian's journey to finding joy

by Adrian Adger

Published by Adrian and Karen Adger

Contact:
Clough Presbyterian Church
18 The Square, Clough, Downpatrick, County Down BT30 8RB

Seaforde Presbyterian Church
Demense Road, Seaforde, Downpatrick, County Down BT30 8SG

www.cloughandseaforde.com

ISBN 978-1-9993270-2-6

First edition 2019

Printed and bound in the UK

Contents

Foreword

Let me introduce a dear friend, Rev Adrian Adger. Adrian is facing a battle with cancer. He is only fifty-six years old—but, two years ago, he developed kidney cancer and was given a bleak diagnosis. The latest news is that the doctors have given up on chemotherapy and are giving him immunotherapy. Despite this, Adrian is standing tall for Jesus—both literally and metaphorically! Literally, because Adrian is six feet, seven and a half inches—and that is tall! But also, and more importantly, metaphorically—because Adrian is standing on the promises of Jesus, trusting Him for each day and trusting Him with his future.

Adrian trained at Belfast Bible College, after which he served with Belfast City Mission for many years. For a short while, he also served with Mission Africa, teaching in a Bible College. He faced many dangers, including threats of kidnapping, while pursuing his passion of getting books to Nigerian pastors. In the process, he inspired Africa Christian Textbooks to start our very popular 'book set' projects. Adrian then returned to further studies in Belfast Bible College and Union Theological College, serving in an assistant role in the Ballyclare Presbyterian congregation. In 2015, he took on the role of minister of two churches—Clough Presbyterian Church and Seaforde Presbyterian Church in County Down, Northern Ireland.

With the agreement of the church, he has taken a short sabbatical for the purpose of writing his story. Meanwhile Adrian is continuing with his ministry, preaching and visiting and having many opportunities to share his faith in the face of difficulties, particularly that of a bleak diagnosis.

Here is what my boss, Rev Dr Paul Bailie, CEO of Mission

Africa (Qua Iboe Fellowship) wrote to supporters and friends recently:

> *Friends, greetings. Our dear friend Revd Adrian Adger has given me his permission to draw your prayerful attention to his health situation. As many will know, Adrian served with distinction and dedication at William Wheatley College in Nigeria, where he gained the love and admiration of all. Tragically, this servant of God is living with a diagnosis of cancer. In recent times, his medical situation has become somewhat worse. I promised him this morning that the Mission Africa family would uphold him in prayer at this difficult time. It is our privilege to have had this man of God within our ranks and Adrian is still very much one of us. Please pray for him diligently, especially that his current medical treatment will benefit him. His faith is as inspirational as ever.*

I wholeheartedly recommend Adrian as 'the real deal': he is a genuine, passionate, warm-hearted, reformed, gospel-centred, pastoral, generous, mission-minded servant of Christ.

Rev Dr Sid Garland, International Director-at-large
Africa Christian Textbooks (ACTS)
April 2019

Chapter 1

Finding out

It was a mild February evening in early 2017. My wife, Karen, and I were at home—just the two of us, just a totally normal evening. Right out of the blue, I had a sharp pain in my side. We had absolutely no idea what it could be. Feeling concerned, we telephoned the Out of Hours emergency number for advice—and they told us a doctor would telephone us back. However, the pain very quickly escalated and so we decided that Karen would drive me to A&E at our local hospital—Daisy Hill Hospital in Newry, County Armagh.

The journey was only about forty minutes but, as we travelled to the hospital, the pain became so intense and so extreme that I genuinely thought I was going to die. As we arrived at the hospital, the pain became so severe that I was sick. A paramedic kindly brought a wheelchair to take me into the accident and emergency unit.

Diagnosis

I was quickly seen by a doctor who administered morphine—and the pain subsided fast. The doctors decided that it was likely to have been a kidney stone that was causing it. We were sent home with more pain relief medication and they said they would contact us the next morning about getting a scan in order to confirm the diagnosis. As the pain eased off, so did our concerns.

The next day, after a few hours' sleep? I woke feeling rather tired.

We hadn't heard anything about the follow-up scan, so we phoned the hospital. They asked us to return. A scan was completed within the hour—and we waited for the results. The doctor told us that the scan had revealed a large tumour in my kidney. As you can imagine, that was a massive shock to me. I had come to terms with the idea of a kidney stone—but the word 'tumour' had not entered my head at that point. It was hard to take in and hard to understand. The consultant said that, at this stage, they did not know if the tumour was malignant or benign—although he did say that it could possibly be cancer. He said that it was likely that I would have an operation to remove the entire kidney. Then he said, 'It looks like we have got it in time.'

So that's exactly what happened. Eight weeks later, in early April, I had an operation at Craigavon Area Hospital, County Armagh to remove my kidney. A month after that, Karen and I went to meet the consultant to talk about the results of the operation. I was apprehensive and I was sick on the way there—primarily from nerves, although the journey didn't help. We waited anxiously in the small waiting area in the renal unit. The consultant was professional, calm and reassuring—and the news was good. Even though the tumour was malignant, the lymph nodes around the kidney were clear so the cancer was confined to the kidney and had not spread.

All clear

No further treatment was required. We travelled home relieved and very happy. I was off work for about ten weeks, recovering from the operation. After that, I was given the 'all clear' and was delighted to continue as a church minister in Clough and Seaforde, County Down.

We were calm and positive as we approached the 'routine' six-monthly scan in October and were quietly confident that everything would be fine. I had a busy weekend teaching God's Word on the Friday evening at an autumn conference for Child Evangelism Fellowship at a local church in County Down. I was also teaching morning and evening on the Sunday at my home churches: Clough and Seaforde Presbyterian. We were not thinking too much about the scan and we were enjoying our ministry and our life together.

Another scan

We went back to Craigavon Hospital to receive the results in early November. The consultant said to me, 'Now this is really out of the blue—I wasn't expecting this.' That wasn't good... There were new lesions in my abdomen—and they were inoperable. I now had incurable cancer. It was an unbelievable shock.

My mind was spinning. It felt like a death sentence coming over me, a dark cloud—like a heavy, heavy burden that I suddenly had to carry. And the thought that kept running round my mind was this: 'Would I ever know joy again in my life?' Karen and I cried all night. We were heartbroken—we just couldn't understand it. We had been married just four years at that point. Apart from God's gift of salvation, Karen is the best thing that has ever happened to me in my life—and we really love one another. We were totally devastated and completely disorientated.

Hopes and dreams

Our hopes and dreams as a couple seemed to go up in smoke. Our hopes and dreams of serving the Lord seemed over. We had been living in County Down for just two years; we felt like round pegs in round holes—completely at home. We were loving the ministry we were involved with—and the incredible love that the people had showed us. Having been here only two years, we felt we were just beginning. New families had been joining both churches and new ministries had been set up. We had just set up our churches' Facebook page, we planned for home groups and new elders. I could not understand it. Why me? Why now? I felt as if I was being cut down in the midst of life. Only fifty-four. I began to wonder whether God was punishing me for something I'd done wrong.

At the beginning of January, I began the chemotherapy treatment. For me, the consultant recommended using a drug called Sutent, which was in tablet form. The consultant in the Cancer Centre in the City Hospital also told us that the results were mixed. In one third of patients, the lesions grew; in one third, the lesions stayed the same; and in one third, there was shrinkage. We realised that whatever happened next was in God's hands. By God's grace, in April, July and October 2018, I had three good scan results. I gather that radiologists do not normally comment on scan results. They made just one comment about my last scan: 'unusual'. Thankfully, I managed to continue with my work and we saw many encouragements over those months.

My next scan was in early January 2019 and I had an appointment booked for Monday 7 January to receive the results. What would 2019 hold for us? Having had three positive scan results, we were hopeful of a fourth. At the same time, I became anxious as we waited for the results. I woke up a few times in the early hours of that Monday morning as I began to feel apprehensive about the scan results later in the day.

Shock

Karen and I travelled to Belfast City Hospital in good time for our afternoon appointment. We waited nervously in the Bridgewater Suite of the Cancer Centre for the result of this next three-monthly scan. The consultant took us along a corridor and we went into a side room with him. He explained that the chemotherapy was no longer working and that the tumours in my abdomen were now growing again. The cancer had also spread from my abdomen to my liver. He was recommending that I should now start a new treatment called immunotherapy.

We were devastated by this latest setback and in shock. We could not take in the fact that the cancer was now growing again after one whole year of positive results. We just didn't expect it. Yet, we were also thankful for the new treatment being offered. We came home and tried to digest the news. We wept and we prayed. How were we going to share more bad news with our family and friends? We began the difficult process of telling family, church and friends—yet again. As I spoke to my immediate family and my closest friend, the tears flowed. We prayed and wept together. I felt thoroughly disorientated.

Now here I am, three months on, living with a grim cancer diagnosis. Nothing has changed—and yet, everything has changed. By God's grace, I have found peace again after being totally disorientated. I have found a new confidence and a new joy. And I can honestly say that I'm excited about what God has for me in the future. How is that possible? I'd love to tell you.

Chapter 2

Finding my feet

First, I must take you back several decades... I was raised in a bungalow on my grandparents' farm near Ballymena, Northern Ireland. My father's parents were called Robert and Elizabeth Adger and their first family home had been in a terraced house on the Russellstown Road, near Galgorm, Ballymena, where they had brought up their seven children: Lily, Mary, Bob, Bella, Frank, William (my father) and Margaret. In 1939, my grandparents bought a nearby farm.

My parents

The first time my father met my mother, Eileen, was at a dance in Halls Hotel in Antrim.[1] They were married in 1956, in Lylehill Presbyterian Church (not far from Antrim) where Eileen used to sing in the church choir. With the help of Bob, Frank and Robert (his two brothers and the husband of his sister, Lily), William built a bungalow on the farm.[2] I was their first child, born on the 9 March 1963. Neil, their second, was born a couple of years later—on 3 November 1965.

The farm had a cow for milking, a loft for pigeons, some chickens for eggs, a donkey called Nellie for playing and a dog called Skippy for walking. The fields were rented out to local farmers for keeping cattle or growing potatoes. I remember gathering potatoes all day for the princely sum of 50 pence! Neil and I would take

1 My father, William Adger was born in 1927. My mother Eileen Mary Cuming was born in 1932.

2 The farm was at 12 Lisnafillon Road. My parents' house was on the farm, at 14 Lisnafillon Road.

Skippy for walks in the nearby fields, along with Martha Ashcroft, one of our neighbours. My father served his apprenticeship as a joiner with Harland & Wolf shipyard in Belfast. He then moved to work with McLoughlin & Harvey's Construction Company and became Contracts Manager. When the County Hall was built outside Ballymena, my father was the Site Manager. My mother devoted her attention to bringing up us two boys. We had a happy childhood. The family also rented a shop in Church Street, Ballymena, called Motherhood, selling maternity and other clothes, which she managed for a number of years.

William and Eileen were occasional attenders of the local church—Trinity Presbyterian Church, Ahoghill—in the early years of their married life. They would have attended services at Harvest, Christmas and Easter. William a keen golfer and, at one stage, was a member of both Ballymena Golf Club and Royal Portrush Golf Club. Sunday was a great day for playing golf! My parents both had good morals. They were honest and they worked hard. Neither of them smoked cigarettes or drank alcohol.

An invitation to Sunday School

One day, a neighbour called Billy Steele, said to my parents that he would be willing to take me to Sunday School at the church. My mother said she would wait until Neil was also old enough to go. And so, some time later, Billy Steele began to collect Neil and me and take us to Sunday School. My father would collect us afterwards and take us home. My parents began to feel uneasy about not taking their children to church themselves, so the four of us began attending Trinity Presbyterian Church together.

Over the next four years, this became their pattern and they heard the gospel being preached by the minister, Dr Harry Uprichard. A colleague of William's from work, Bob Brown, also began to talk to him about the Christian faith. One day, my father brought home some booklets about the Christian gospel and left them in the living room. My mother was not at all pleased about this! She said to her husband that if he wanted to give his life to the Lord, she certainly would not be following suit! Eileen felt William was trying to push her in a direction she really did not want to go.

The seeds of faith

Although she was not aware of it at the time, the Lord was speaking to Eileen. Eventually, in 1972, Eileen knew that all was not well between her and God and that she urgently needed to do something about it. She called to speak to the minister at his home—the 'manse'. Dr Uprichard explained the good news of Jesus Christ to her: he told her that Jesus Christ had come into the world with a purpose in mind—to save sinners. That same day, Eileen repented of her sin and believed in the Lord Jesus Christ and was saved by God's grace (Ephesians 2:8-9). Eileen said that her experience of salvation was like taking a bath and the stains of sin being removed. She came out of the bath feeling completely clean for the first time in her life.

William came home from work that same day and took the two boys to the Boys Brigade (an international, interdenominational Christian youth organisation in Northern Ireland and other countries). As he returned home, he was wondering whether to call at the Knowles family for some eggs, or whether to call at the minister's house instead? He decided to visit the minister and he too believed in the Lord Jesus Christ and was born again of the Spirit of God. A tremendous change took place in their lives and they had a new passion to live a life to please the Lord, their new Master (2 Corinthians 5:17).

A new pattern

William never played golf on a Sunday again. Sunday became a day for going to church with the family, both in the morning and the evening. It was always Trinity Presbyterian Church in the morning. And, in the evening, the services rotated between three churches: First Ahoghill Presbyterian, Brookside Presbyterian Church and Trinity Presbyterian Church. They attended church with a new sense of purpose to worship God their Creator, Saviour and Shepherd. At home, there were also changes. William would now gather the family around the Bible to read and share God's good news with us children. Prayers and praise were offered to God as we gathered together in the kitchen. Before every meal was eaten, William would now say grace, giving thanks to the Lord for providing food for another day.

Now no television was allowed on a Sunday, which was known as 'The Lord's Day' and was different from all the other days of the week. I remember this particularly as my favourite programme was 'The Golden Shot' which was hosted by Bob Monkhouse—on a Sunday. I was no longer allowed to watch 'The Golden Shot'—and there was no 'catch-up' television in those days! I was not happy at first, but I quickly accepted the new norm. Sunday afternoons as a family were now enjoyed by going for a walk in the countryside. Appreciating the outdoors and the beauty of the God's creation became important. I loved all this and we built many good memories.

Childhood wrongdoing

I am not sure that our attendance at church had much of an impact on my behaviour as a small boy. I had not grasped the truth and, naturally, I was going my own way in life. Neil and I attended the local Gracehill Primary School, just like William and other members of the Adger family before us. I came home from Gracehill Primary one day and said a 'bad word' that I had heard at school, in front of my mum. Despite trying to run to another room in the house, mum ensured I was lovingly disciplined and that she taught me what was right and wrong.

Another day, I remember feeling hungry, so decided to reach up and take a bite of an apple on the tree in the garden. Afterwards, I ran into the house and was sitting with Neil at the kitchen table. Mum came in and asked which one of us had eaten from the apple tree. I immediately denied it, then mum asked again. I said. 'It was Neil'. Mum looked straight at me and said, 'Why are your teeth marks on the apple?' A mother's instinct? Whatever it was, I was found out.[3]

In the final year of primary school, I was sitting beside Hazel McKendry in class. Hazel was much better at spellings than I ever was, so, if I wasn't sure of an answer, I had a 'juke over' to see Hazel's answer. One day, Hazel spelt one of her spellings wrong. She had mixed up the 'a' and 'u' of the word 'guard'. Guess who also spelt the word 'guard' wrong? That is right... me. After the spelling test was handed in, our teacher Mr Coulter came to our table and asked us, 'Which one of you is copying?' My face went bright red and I knew I was found out.

---

3 Numbers 32:23

Chapter 3

Finding forgiveness

After Gracehill Primary, I went on to grammar school at Ballymena Academy and I enjoyed my time there. I took a keen interest in football and could often be found playing football at lunchtime in the school playground. I also began to watch Ballymena United Football club at the Ballymena Showgrounds on a Saturday afternoon. Once, John Sloan—who played for Ballymena FC—came into school to talk about his Christian faith. That was the only time I ever attended the Scripture Union Christian meeting!

Teenage struggles

As I grew older, I began to swear more and more. It became so bad that I could not use many sentences without a swear word included. Later, like so many teenagers, I also began to drink alcohol. A group of us would hang out at The Countryman pub in Ballymena and drink there. There were also times that I bought alcohol at a local off-licence and got drunk. My behaviour was deteriorating. On Saturday evenings, I used to go to the local disco in the nearby Tullyglass Hotel. In 1981, at the age of 18, I passed my A Levels and left home to study accountancy at Stirling University in Scotland. Mathematics was my best subject—and I had a strong desire to pursue a career in the accountancy profession. I was motivated to succeed and I was pleased to be gaining my independence.

Around this time, I decided that church was dull and boring—so I stopped going. I wanted to enjoy myself and I didn't want any rules or regulations. Religion was not relevant to my life in any way. To my shame, at university, along with others, I would sometimes get so drunk at the weekend that I could only stagger home to my halls of residence. Socialising and drinking alcohol were becoming more and more important to me and my studies suffered as a result. Despite this, I managed to graduate in 1984 with a degree in Accountancy from the university.

All change

At this point, I had no intention of returning to Northern Ireland as I planned to continue my accountancy training at a college in Edinburgh. However, the entrance requirements for the course changed, so I had little choice but to go home to the village of Ahoghill. Reluctantly, I returned home to Northern Ireland and studied at University of Ulster at the Jordanstown campus, completing a Diploma in Financial accountancy. It was hard work but I enjoyed living on campus and making new friends. After an interview, I agreed to sign a contract to become a trainee chartered accountant with Deloitte Haskins & Sells at their office in High Street, Belfast. Within a few weeks of moving to Belfast to live and work, my life was about to take a dramatic change.

One evening, I was driving, on my own, to Tracks nightclub in Portrush. I was twenty-two years old and it was around dusk. Suddenly, there was a tractor right in front of me, travelling incredibly slowly, and I had to swerve onto the wrong side of the road to miss it. Immediately, I saw an enormous lorry hurtling towards me—and I had to swerve back again to miss the lorry. I almost died that night, on the Coleraine to Portrush road. It really shook me up.

A few days later, on Wednesday 18 September 1985, I woke up in the morning and I was gasping to breathe. I thought it must be a heart attack and I was desperately afraid. A friend rushed me by car to the City Hospital. The doctor diagnosed that I had experienced a panic attack, possibly brought on by the near car accident or the stress of beginning a new job in Belfast. I was admitted to the hospital and, as I lay on the bed, I felt desperately alone and very shaken by the whole episode.

What if I die today?

I found myself asking the question: 'If I die today, where I would be going?' My first thought was, 'I have absolutely no chance of going to heaven. I was drunk at the weekend and have been living totally for myself.' Then I thought, 'If I am not going to heaven, then where else would I go?' For the first time in my life, I began to think about hell. I became desperately afraid of dying as I knew I was on the wrong road in life and that hell was my destination. I became really alarmed.

I was discharged from the hospital that afternoon and decided I needed to travel home to the comfort of my parents. As I drove out of Belfast on the motorway, I began to think about my life—which was an absolute mess. My life was going downhill very fast and I realised that I hated the way I was living. I wondered how God could ever forgive someone like me. It just didn't seem possible that he could.

Wholehearted prayers

Then I remembered a prayer that I had been taught in Sunday school.

Come into my life, Lord Jesus,
come in today,
come in to stay,
come into my life, Lord Jesus.

As I was driving my car, I prayed that prayer. I wanted to make sure—so I prayed it again. Tears began to flow down my cheeks, and I felt broken. Instantly, I became aware that the Lord Jesus was alive. I knew he had heard my despairing cry—but I realised that, at the same time, the devil had a grip on my life. I returned home and shared my story with my parents. My father, William, said to me, 'Son, that is the best decision you have ever made in your life. Others will let you down, but the Lord will never let you down.' My mother asked me if I wanted to see the minister. I said that I did and went to the manse to talk to him.

Dr Harry Uprichard, who had also been the minister when I was a boy, explained the need to repent and turn away from my sin. He then explained the significance of Jesus' death on the cross. I had heard about the cross at Calvary many times before—but it had never made sense and it all seemed to go over my head. However, this time it was totally different. Dr Uprichard explained that God really loved *me*, and that Jesus had died in *my* place, taking the punishment *my* sins deserved. It was now so clear to me.[4] I could hardly understand or take in what the Lord Jesus had done for me.

With new understanding, I prayed again asking Jesus for forgiveness, asking Him to take complete control of my life and thanking Him for His great salvation. I immediately felt the burden of my own guilt was taken away—the burden that I had been carrying myself up until then. I was so full of joy—I felt like I was walking in the clouds. I knew for the first time in my life that I could place my head on my pillow that evening and not be afraid of death anymore because I had the certainty that I was on my way to heaven. *Hallelujah.*

New joy

I travelled back to Belfast with a spring in my step. That evening, I opened my Bible which I had not read for a number of years. The first verse that really struck me was from 1 John 3:8—'The reason the Son of God appeared was to destroy the devil's work.' I knew that the Son of God had come to destroy the devil's work in my life.

A member of my home church came to see me and invited me to join a group going to hear Derick Bingham teach the Bible. And, the following Sunday, I returned to Trinity Presbyterian Church, Ahoghill—the church of my childhood. The welcome I received

4 1 Peter 3:18

was amazing. John Shaw, among others, shook my hand at the door to express his love for me and gratitude to the Lord Jesus and I was accepted back into the church family with open arms.

I had found a spiritual home where I could learn more about my new faith and grow spiritually. I quickly discovered that the problem had not been with my church—but with my bad attitude towards it, which I repented of. Within a few weeks, there was a meeting after church about starting up a youth fellowship for the first time. I ended up being chosen as one of the leaders, along with a close friend—Martin Dickey. We would serve together in the youth fellowship on a Sunday evening for the next nine years. I also had the privilege of teaching children in the Sunday school which I loved.

Humiliation

After a few years, I started receiving invitations to speak in other youth fellowships. On one particular Sunday evening, I was speaking at a youth fellowship in a church in Ballymena. I had made some notes and I put them in front of me, on the lectern. Part-way through the message I was preaching, I went 'off-script'. When I stopped and looked down at my notes, I had no idea where I was in my notes. After a long pause, I regained my place and continued preaching.

Afterwards, a friend said to me that he'd really felt for me in my embarrassment. I was so discouraged and disheartened. I told myself that I never wanted to preach, ever again! I spent much of the next day in work thinking that I never wanted to make a fool of myself like that again—and that I was finished with preaching! Then I suddenly remembered that I was due to speak in the youth fellowship at Trinity in the very near future... I couldn't let them down. By God's grace, that went well—so I was back up on my feet and serving again. I also decided to use fewer notes in speaking, hoping that would give me more freedom.

New priorities

I continued working as an accountant for Deloitte Haskins & Sells. Alongside my day-to-day work, I had professional accountancy examinations to complete. The best available preparation course operated over a number of Saturdays and Sundays. I had a decision to make. What was more important—my accountancy exams or getting to church each week?

I decided to enrol on a different course which allowed me to be in church every Sunday. I successfully passed some of the professional examinations but failed the final examination to become a chartered accountant. The disappointment did not last long as I felt the Lord was at work in my life.

One day, one of the managers in my firm looked out of the window of the third-floor High Street office block, gazing over the Belfast horizon. There had been terrorist murders in the city and a lot of suffering. He walked over to me and asked me, 'Is there any God out there?' I remember replying, 'Yes, there is. I was talking to Him this morning!' I knew I did not understand everything, but I knew enough to be sure that the Lord was alive and active in the world.

A close shave

While working at Deloitte Haskins & Sells, I moved house to live in South Belfast. In mid-December 1986, there was a knock at the door. It was close to midnight. Trevor Gage (my landlord and housemate) answered the door. An RUC (Royal Ulster Constabulary) policeman said that there was a bomb around the corner. We needed to evacuate the house immediately.

We left straightaway. Minutes later, I walked through the door of the Belfast City Mission Hall in Great Northern Street. When the bomb exploded, there was a rush of wind down the street. The 600lb bomb totally demolished Lisburn Road RUC Station—my room had overlooked it. At 4.30 am, when we were allowed back into the house, I inspected my room. The glass from the window was in the far corner of the room. The curtains and the poles had been blasted to the other side. If I had been sitting at the table, would I have survived the bomb blast? It was a close shave.

That night, I slept in another room in the house and, later that morning, travelled into work. Many suffered as a result of the bombing perpetrated by the IRA: seven people were injured, 800 homes and scores of business premises were damaged, and the Evangelical Presbyterian Church building was completely destroyed. But it was clear that the Lord still had plans and purposes for my life.

A new direction

Through reading God's Word, I felt I was being led away from the accountancy firm to serve in the Republic of Ireland with European Christian Mission for three months in the summer of 1990. Christian mission was becoming a greater passion in my life and more important to me than being an accountant. That decision met with various different reactions... One person said to me, 'You are mad to be leaving an accountancy career to do that.' Personally, I felt I would be mad not to! To me, this was simply a step of obedience to Scripture.

After nearly five years in Cooper & Lybrand Deloitte (as the firm became known), the staff kindly came together and gave me a good send-off. With the gift of money they gave me, I bought as many commentaries as possible from a local Christian bookshop. I also bought recordings of some talks by a pastor called Willie Mullan and I used to listen to them while travelling in the car. My desire to learn from the Scriptures was growing.[5]

I had a tremendous time in the summer with the European Christian Mission, serving in Dublin, Clonmel and Dungarvan, speaking at open air meetings in churches and doing door-to-door visits, speaking to people about the Christian faith. My faith in the Lord was being strengthened by this short-term mission trip.

---

5 1 Peter 2:2-3

When I returned home to Ahoghill, I had no plans but I began to help my father with a new business he had set up called 'Trend Cards'. He had a card stand built for the back of a van and he sold packs of greeting cards to shops throughout Northern Ireland. Then a local businessman, William Wright, suggested that I should join his family-run company—Robert Wright & Son (coach works) in Galgorm—to help prepare for the annual audit that was coming up. So, I worked part-time in the accountancy department of the company for some months. God was showing his love in providentially guiding me and providing for me. And God had other plans that were about to be revealed!

Chapter 4

FINDING GUIDANCE

Although I didn't always know what the next step in my life would be, God did—and, step by step, His plan for my life unfolded. The Lord has led me by His Word, by His Spirit and through the wise counsel of friends. He has closed some doors and opened other doors of opportunity. I continued to attend Trinity Presbyterian Church regularly. The minister taught faithfully through God's Word—and his expository preaching ministry was strengthening me in my faith.

The doctrines of grace and the reformed faith with its emphasis on the sovereignty of God were stirring my heart. Those great truths that were rediscovered during the sixteenth century Reformation—that salvation is by Scripture alone, by faith alone, through Christ alone, and to the glory of God alone—were now becoming very important to me.

God's call

One Wednesday evening, I was at the church midweek meeting. A missionary from World Evangelisation Crusade was speaking. He had planned to travel to the country of Macedonia in Europe in order to share the gospel. He was speaking from Acts 16:9 where the apostle Paul has a vision of a man of Macedonia standing and begging him, 'Come over to Macedonia and help us.' Paul and the ministry team then left for Macedonia, concluding that God had called them to preach the gospel there. As I listened to the missionary, I knew that message was just for me. The Lord was now calling me to leave and travel to a 'Macedonia' to preach the gospel there. I wasn't yet sure where that would be—but I felt sure that He wanted me to do it.

I became aware that I knew so little about the Bible and that I needed to be further equipped in ministry. So I applied to study for three years at Belfast Bible College at Dunmurray and was accepted to begin in September 1991. At the welcome weekend retreat, I met Brian and Pamela Smyth. Little did I know how significant this friendship would be in my life. In the first semester, Brian and I became part of a prayer triplet together.

Stepping out

During the second year of studies, everyone was required to complete an overseas placement for two months. I had planned to travel to Israel for my placement—but, one evening, I was invited to First Ahoghill Presbyterian Church to hear about the work of some missionaries from Asia. An appeal for workers was made and I stood up and dedicated myself to serve the Lord. As I left the meeting, it was the country of Kenya that was in my mind—although Kenya wasn't even mentioned at the meeting! But I believe the Spirit was now directing me to travel to the continent of Africa for the first time.

I was directed towards AIM International and plans were made for me to visit an area in the North of Kenya where I would stay with a missionary family called the Barfoots from Scotland. At first, I was really looking forward to travelling there. However, I soon became much more aware of all the difficulties. I was going to an area with a high risk for malaria. Then I read in the local press about someone dying from malaria, as well as a volunteer with the mission being killed in tribal clashes. I then read from Revelation 2:10, 'Do not be afraid about what you are about to suffer.' I concentrated on the phrase 'about to suffer'—rather than the 'Do not be afraid'! Looking at all these things together, I became desperately afraid and I worried that some calamity was going to befall me.

On the Sunday before I was due to fly to Nairobi, I was at Trinity Presbyterian and Kenneth Scullion preached from the Gospels on the passage in which Peter stepped out of the boat and walked on the water of the Sea of Galilee (Matthew 14:22-34). But then he looked around at the storm, became afraid, and began to sink into the water. After Peter called out, Jesus lifted him up and rescued him, as well as challenging him about his little faith and doubt. I identified with Peter that morning and I knew I was sinking fast, spiritually speaking, but I was comforted in knowing that Jesus was there to provide all the help that was needed. Strengthened by God's Word, I travelled to Kenya—knowing I was not alone. The short-term mission trip turned out to be a great blessing and my fears were groundless.

Discovering my limitations

Sometimes it was a question of being guided not to do something! There was a choir at Belfast Bible College and I joined them for practices. However, at one rehearsal, the choir mistress said that some people were not hitting the right notes, and would we mind if she pointed out the culprits. You may guess what happened next... The lady came over to me and I was asked to leave the choir! The next day, I received a small Mars bar in my pigeon hole, along with a note which said: 'Cheer up you haven't been thrown out of the heavenly choir.' It is good to know our limitations as well as our gifts!

Towards the end of my three-year Diploma in Theology course, I wondered what ministry I should be involved in next. I considered a position as a youth and community worker in Ballysally Presbyterian Church in Coleraine, near the north coast of Northern Ireland, about fifty-five miles from Belfast. At first, I wasn't very keen to apply since I didn't know anyone in Coleraine. Soon after, I met a lady at Belfast Bible College who was planning to travel to China. I felt rebuked by her faith and courage especially as I was unwilling to travel to Coleraine! I decided to apply—but I was then turned down after an interview. I then applied for another job—but this time I did not even receive an interview. Someone then asked me why I hadn't got a job yet. I felt very discouraged. I had given up a good accountancy career and nothing seemed to be working out for me.

New challenges

In September 1994, my best friend Brian Smyth told me about a vacancy in one of the inner-city districts served by the Belfast City Mission (BCM). Belfast City Mission is an urban mission which has been involved in community evangelism on the streets of Belfast for over 190 years. At present, they cover sixteen districts where they have Mission Halls and centres used for evangelism. Brian had recently begun serving in one of the BCM districts in North Belfast. I thought and prayed about this opportunity for a few months. Brian asked me to speak at his first Harvest service in Mountcollyer Mission Hall and took me on some door-to-door visitation in North Belfast. I talked with the Assistant Secretary and Executive Secretary of BCM—Robin Fairbairn and George Ferguson—because I wanted to make as informed a decision as possible.

As I wrestled with this decision, the Lord spoke to me through the words he spoke to Paul in Acts 18:9-10. 'Do not be afraid; keep on speaking, do not be silent. For I am with you, and no-one is going to attack and harm you, because I have many people in this city.' I decided to fill in the application form. The day I posted it, I experienced a tremendous sense of peace. The Lord had called me to this ministry. I was interviewed by the Board of BCM and completed my trial sermon at Ballysillan Hall in North Belfast. I was accepted to be a missionary with BCM and I was posted to a new work at the Woodvale Mission Hall in Disraeli Street in the Upper Shankill area of North Belfast.

Serving in the Woodvale Mission Hall

My first meeting at the Woodvale took place at the beginning of December 1994. I was very discouraged. Coming from the countryside into the Shankill, there were certainly differences in culture. There was no pianist, so I had been given an unfamiliar red-coloured

Redemption Hymnal and was leading the singing with my 'not-great' singing voice (remember my experience in the choir!). There were twelve people in the meeting. I asked myself whether I had made a mistake. The following Sunday morning, my home congregation held a commissioning service for me and Dr Uprichard preached. The elders laid their hands on me, I left the service fully assured that the Lord was with me and knowing that was enough.

In January 1995, I called in to visit a lady who had come to the Mission Hall a few times. She told me she was a Mormon and had been baptised into the Mormon Church. I said to her: 'Let's read from the Bible.' She ran upstairs to get her Mormon Bible. When she came downstairs, I said to her, 'You know what you can do with that?' 'What?' she replied and I said, 'Throw it in the fire, for it's of no use to you.' To my surprise, she threw her Bible into the open fire in the living room and she knelt down on her knees on the floor and asked the Lord Jesus to be her Saviour and Lord. She stopped any friendship with the Mormons and she committed herself to come to the Hall. That was a further confirmation from the Lord that I was doing His will.

One Sunday morning, I woke up early. I was due to speak at two country churches and I was worried because I felt I had the wrong message for them. So I decided instead to speak on Jesus calming the storm, from Matthew 14. At the end of the service, a couple came up to speak to me. The lady said she had recently been diagnosed with cancer and that she had an operation to go through, followed by chemotherapy. She said that the message had been just for her. It is true that, if we are listening, we are able to hear the voice of Jesus in any storm.

During my time in the Woodvale Mission Hall, Brian Smyth and I were asked to conduct a week-long gospel mission in Aughantaine Presbyterian Church outside Fivemiletown, County Tyrone, on behalf of the Belfast City Mission. There were meetings in the evening and visits during the afternoon. The Spirit of God was at work and four people professed faith in Jesus Christ during that time. One older man who was a farmer said to us that he had given his life to the Lord on the Tuesday—and that it was the best day of his life! One young woman was broken and wept tears of repentance. The Lord continued to guide me while I served at BCM.

Changes

Over the years, there were inevitable changes—missionaries (including Brian) moved to other ministries. In June 2000, I moved within BCM to serve in the Fairview Road Hall, Newtownabbey (about ten miles north of Belfast). I had a wonderful time there. During the years, a good news club ceased and a youth club, mission support group, praise group, mother and toddlers and discipleship group were started up. Leslie Reid from Dungannon came alongside to assist in the ministry for some years. I also took on the role of Mayor's chaplain for Victor Robinson, reading the Scriptures and leading in prayer at the beginning of the council meetings.

My mum

In March 2004, I visited my mum in the Royal Victoria Hospital in Belfast. By God's grace, my mum was saved when she was forty years old. However, when she was just sixty-five years old, she was diagnosed with Alzheimer's. Over the years, it robbed her of her memory and her personality. On this particular visit, I quoted the words of my mum's favourite hymn that she had learned when she was a girl.

When the trumpet of the Lord shall sound,
And time shall be no more,
And the morning breaks, eternal, bright and fair;
When the saved of earth shall gather
Over on the other shore,
And the roll is called up yonder... [6]

6 James M Black, 'When the Roll is Called Up Yonder', 1893.

Mum then looked up and lifted her hand up to point upwards. And she said, 'I'll be there.' The last line of the hymn. It was an incredible moment. Despite her debilitating illness, she knew where she was going.

The worst Christmas

A short time later, my mum was discharged from the hospital. On Christmas Day that year, I received a telephone call from my father at 7.45 am in the morning. My father told me that my mother's breathing was laboured but that he had called an ambulance. At 8.10 am, I received another call to say that mum had passed away. That was an enormous shock. I prepared to make my way home. I came out of the house and there was snow on the ground. My neighbour called out 'Happy Christmas' to me. He meant well—but little did he know that it was the worst Christmas of my life and that I was still in a state of bewilderment.

But the Lord comforted us through our friends and His Word. I will never forget Billy and Mary Steele kindly providing food for us when we did not feel like cooking. My brother Neil, and our family and friends gathered for the service in the home a few days later. Dr Harry Uprichard gave an uplifting address.

Hope amid the grief

The burial took place at the family grave plot in Trinity Presbyterian Church graveyard. I was still heartbroken, distressed and sorrowing. I always feel that going to the graveyard with the coffin is the hardest part of all, due to the finality of death. Yet that day, the word 'hope' came to my mind. I realised afresh that these were only my mother's mortal remains. My mother was not going into the grave—because she was already singing in the heavenly choir.

A few days earlier, when my mum breathed her last in the family home in Lisnafillon Road, angels came and carried her soul to Abraham's side. Now my father didn't see any angels as he attended her—but I am in no doubt that they were there, just as angels carried the beggar, Lazarus, to the Abraham's side in Luke 16:22. I was given new hope. I grieved deeply for my mum, but I didn't grieve without hope (1 Thessalonians 4:13). The trumpet would sound one day and there would be a great reunion of God's people (1 Thessalonians 4:16).

A place of darkness

On one occasion, I needed a minor hernia operation. It seemed to be a routine procedure and I was not concerned about it at all. The operation was successful but the recovery process was more difficult. While I was convalescing at home, I was often emotional and had no idea why tears came so readily. I was low in spirit as I sought to move forward in life. A few days later, I took some medication during the night and a cloud of darkness came over my mind. I found myself in a dark place I had never been before and was desperately afraid and anxious. I talked to my father who was sympathetic and supportive but was unable to understand my dilemma. I could not understand why darkness seemed to envelop me and I felt I had nothing to look forward to in life.

I needed someone to help. Who could I turn to? I telephoned a Christian counsellor I knew and she said I needed to make an appointment with the doctor. That was the best advice I could ever have received. My family doctor was tremendously understanding and he listened before giving me expert medical advice. I needed a prescription of sleeping tablets as I was not sleeping well. He also prescribed me some antidepressants. The medication was necessary in my recovery and was used by the Lord to strengthen me. After a number of weeks, I was able to return to work. My confidence had been shaken but it gradually returned. I visited a Christian counsellor for around some months who gave me wise counsel in handling the difficulties I had experienced. After the course of antidepressants, I was fully restored.

The Scriptures were an enormous comfort and in particular the Psalms, especially Psalm 18:28-29:

> *You, Lord, keep my lamp burning;*
> *my God turns my darkness into light.*
> *With your help I can advance against a troop;*
> *with my God I can scale a wall.*

Why did I go through that experience? There are no easy answers—yet, at the same time, 2 Corinthians 1:3-4 provides an important perspective:

> *Praise be to the God and Father of our Lord Jesus Christ, the Father of compassion and the God of all comfort, who comforts us in all our troubles, so that we can comfort those in any trouble with the comfort we ourselves receive from God.*

I give thanks to my Father in heaven who was so compassionate towards me when I was at my weakest and lowest. God comforted, consoled, strengthened, helped, refreshed and guided me through that time of trouble so that I might be a comfort to others in their time of adversity.

Chapter 5

Finding inspiration in Africa

Monday 2 April 2007 was just another day in my life, or was it? I had driven to Ballymoney, County Antrim, to be involved in an evangelism team for a mission that Belfast City Mission (BCM) were conducting in the town. That day, a colleague called Paul Hamill asked me if I would like to join him in travelling to Burkina Faso for two weeks in the summer for a mission trip. I found it so challenging that he was using some of his holidays to serve the Lord in Africa. I had never thought of doing that before. I began to pray and ask the Lord if He wanted me to travel there.

Off to Africa

The country of Nigeria came to mind, because the people in the Mission Hall followed the work of Pamela Johnston. Pamela is a missionary in Jos with Mission Africa. (In September 2008, Pamela married Professor Musa Gaiya, a widower from Jos. The wedding was in Belfast and I had the privilege of attending—it was a wonderful day.) On the Tuesday morning, I had no idea what I should do next. I prayed, 'Lord, please show me what you want me to do by next Tuesday.'

The next thing that happened was that I was asked by the new Executive Secretary of BCM, Bobi Brown, to lead two church services in July—at exactly the same time as the Burkina Faso mission trip. So that door was firmly closed. I decided to contact Pamela. She replied that there were opportunities to speak at a theological college and in churches. I felt very afraid and inadequate. I could never do anything like that. It was way beyond me. It seemed impossible.

One Saturday evening, I heard a man from the New Tribes Mission speaking from the book of Haggai. He mentioned Haggai 2:4-5.

> *'Be strong ... and work. For I am with you,' declares the Lord Almighty ... 'And my Spirit remains among you. Do not fear.'*

I felt reassured. On the following Tuesday, I was in Bangor at the Faith Mission Easter Convention. John Brand of Africa Inland Mission International was speaking on Matthew 9:37-38.

> *Then he said to his disciples, 'The harvest is plentiful but the workers are few. Ask the Lord of the harvest, therefore, to send out workers into his harvest field.'*

Broken before the Lord

John Brand challenged those of us present about using two or three weeks of our holidays to be involved in a mission trip. I was in tears, I was broken before the Lord. Then he said, 'It is not *ability*, but *availability* that counts.' I said to the Lord, 'I don't have much to give but I am available.' I contacted Mission Africa and Chief Executive, Paul Bailie, recommended that I spend one week in the north of Nigeria (in Jos) and two weeks in the south (at the William Wheatley Theological College). The Vice Provost of the College in Nigeria, Rev O P Jonah, was studying at Belfast Bible College at that time. I arranged to meet him and he said to me that the College in Nigeria had been asking help from Mission Africa for some time! It all sounded very straightforward.

Too tall to keep a low profile

I had contemplated flying into Port Harcourt in the Niger Delta but was advised that there were security issues in the Niger Delta with kidnappings going on. I was told to keep a low profile. It is rather difficult to keep a low profile when you are 6 feet and 7½ inches tall! I was also informed that it would be hot and humid in the south.

I asked Campbell Hamilton, a former missionary in Nigeria, how to prepare for that. He replied, 'Try going into a sauna with your clothes on!' Then I talked to a man who explained to me the dangers of the roads. When he had been in Nigeria, travelling in a car in the evening, they had reached the top of a hill and, at this point, they met a lorry on the wrong side of the road. The driver of their car had to swerve to avoid a head-on collision. I became more aware of the potential difficulties of the mission trip and my faith began to falter. I read from Acts 20.

> *And now, compelled by the Spirit, I am going to … not knowing what will happen to me there … However, I consider my life nothing to me; my only aim is to finish the race and complete the task the Lord Jesus has given me—the task of testifying to the gospel of God's grace.*
>
> (*Acts 20:22, 24*)

Confidence from God's Word

Once again, God's Word gave me the conviction I needed to move forward in confidence and faith. On 22 October 2007, I boarded an aeroplane at the George Best Belfast City Airport to begin a three-week mission trip in Nigeria. During my first week, I enjoyed staying with Professor Musa Gaiya and his sons in Jos in Plateau State in the north of Nigeria. Pamela kindly showed me round her office and helpfully explained more to me about the work of Africa Christian Textbooks (ACTS).

This ministry began when Rev Dr Sid Garland, a lecturer in the

Theological College of Northern Nigeria saw the thirst for books among theological students and lecturers and began shipping books by post from the UK. The ministry developed and now fourteen bookshops have established mostly in theological colleges across Nigeria with the aim of supplying Africans with serious literature at affordable prices. ACTS also encourages African writers to write for their own communities. Students and pastors in Nigeria and also Kenya are being helped through this strategic ministry.

Most of my time in Nigeria was spent at William Wheatley Theological College in the rural Niger Delta. I stayed with Rufus and Iris Ogbonna. Rufus is a minister in the United Evangelical Church and Iris a missionary from Scotland. Both were involved in the life of the College. They were both so kind and hospitable, and they helped me to begin to adapt to a new culture.

Zeal and enthusiasm

The College was founded in 1996 and had seventy full-time students. The majority are already preachers or pastors of churches but they were attending for theological education. Their zeal and enthusiasm was inspiring. Each week, there was an all-night prayer meeting and the students would regularly fast and pray. There was also a real sense of dependence on the Lord in spite of limited resources. The electricity supply was intermittent and, each day, washing was carried out using a bucket of water. When I arrived at the College, I was humbled and moved to tears when I saw their joy as they sang praises to the Lord in song. Their kindness and hospitality were amazing. One of the students said to me, 'I don't have much but here are four apples for your journey home.'

During my visit, I met up with Rev O P Jonah again who was most helpful. There were many opportunities to teach God's Word and, with the Lord's help, I gave twenty lectures on Nehemiah, 2 Timothy and the Trinity. I had opportunities to speak in five different churches including one where there were over 800 people present. After one church service, a lady came up to me holding a live rooster by the legs. I asked the interpreter what I should do with it. He replied that someone would bring it home for me. So it was left in the back of our truck. The next day, it was killed and we had chicken for dinner!

I also spoke at a youth camp and some children's meetings. When one children's meeting was over, the interpreter said to the children, 'You have heard God's message, what are you going to do about it? You need to seek the Lord.' The children began to pray and one six-year-old girl was down on her knees on the concrete floor, with her two hands together, crying out to the Lord.

When I returned home, I knew that the Nigerian believers had had a much more powerful impact on my life than I had ever done on theirs. Back in the Fairview Road Hall of Belfast City Mission, we were able to help the College by providing a new generator. A new partnership in the gospel with our brothers and sisters in Nigeria had begun.

Partnership in the gospel

The following year, 2008, Jonny Beggs (who was on the staff of Mission Africa) asked me about leading a team to William Wheatley Theological College (WWTC) and, as we prayed about it, a 'Go Serve' team came together.

A great team assembled—my best friend Brian and his son Matthew; my good friend Mark Donnelly; Steve Downe from London City Mission; and Heather Gordon from Scotland. We travelled to the College in May 2009 and we gave lectures, spoke at morning meetings to begin the day at WWTC, and taught at children's meetings and in nearby churches.

When I returned home after that three-week mission trip in May 2009, I had no plans to leave the Belfast City Mission or to return to Nigeria. Yet everything changed when I attended the Mission Africa Conference in June of that year. Liam Hanna, a former missionary, spoke at the conference.

He quoted from Exodus 4:2.

> *Then the Lord said to him (Moses), 'What is that in your hand?' 'A staff,' he replied.*

It reminded me of a story of popular author, Belfast pastor and friend Derick Bingham. He was walking along the Lisburn Road in Belfast and the Lord spoke to him, saying, 'What is that in your hand?' Derick looked and he had a pen in his hand so he gave himself to a writing ministry. He went on to write about thirty-five books. I looked at what was in my hand: a Bible.

Two further conversations confirmed to me that the Lord had placed it on my heart to serve at the theological college for six months. The suddenness of God's call shook me to my core. I was taken completely by surprise. I was approaching fifteen years of service in BCM, which I loved. Should I really leave now? Was this some kind of foolish idea that I'd had, which was utterly unrealistic? Was it really of the Lord or not? On Sunday 12 July, I prayed, 'Lord speak to me this evening.' After the meeting at the Fairview Road Hall, we held a prayer meeting and a Polish lady shared Amos 7:14-15.

> *Amos answered Amaziah, 'I was neither a prophet nor the son of a prophet, but I was a shepherd, and I also took care of sycamore-fig trees. But the Lord took me from tending the flock and said to me, "Go, prophesy to my people Israel."'*

There was nothing special about Amos or his family or his background or his education or his job. Amos did not have any special training. What qualified Amos to speak at Bethel? 'The Lord took me ... and said ... "Go."' I sensed that the Lord was taking hold of my life and saying, 'Go to Nigeria' despite my feeling of great inadequacy. On Thursday 6 August, I was driving to meet Paul Bailie, Chief Executive of Mission Africa. I was listening to a CD of some of my favourite worship songs. Suddenly, I felt broken before the Lord and I prayed for His will be done, not mine. Having met with Paul Bailie, he gave a favourable response for me spending six months at WWTC. The Lord had opened a door.

So, on September 2009, I left Belfast City Mission Fairview Road Hall with a heavy heart. The people had shown much love to my father, my late mother and to myself over the years. I was also sorry to leave my colleagues in the Mission. Yet I was leaving at the call of God—and obedience is always paramount. Acts 1:8 came to mind.

> *But you will receive power when the Holy Spirit comes on you; and you will be my witnesses in Jerusalem, and in all Judea and Samaria, and to the ends of the earth.*

Despite my doubts, fears and faltering steps of faith, I was seeking in some way to be a witness for Jesus Christ.

Serving in Nigeria

I left a snowy Northern Ireland for the humid conditions of the Niger Delta at the beginning of January 2010. I was staying in the same compound as Rufus and Iris Ogbonna who were a tremendous support. I was lecturing at the college on three subjects: church growth, the book of Jeremiah, and New Testament survey. Rev Dr Sid Garland helped me prepare for these lectures with his wide experience of lecturing in a Nigerian context.

On the 2009 mission trip, I had become acutely aware of the zeal and thirst that the pastors have for God. Yet, at times, there is a lack of training and resources. There is a dearth of good theological books. The average pastor has few books to help him to teach God's Word—some only have the Bible and very few other books. We discussed about supplying English Standard Study Bibles to every student and lecturer at WWTC and also a collection of other books to form a book set.

The Lord was in this mission trip. I needed to raise over £3,000 for flights, insurance, food, etc. But £11,000 was provided due to the generosity of so many! I was able to use the extra finance raised to help those in need with fees, but especially with books. Sid ordered the ESV Study Bibles in the USA. However, there was one delay after another. The students were praying fervently that the Study Bibles would arrive before I returned home. Finally, in the last week, we received news that they were now on the way and that we would receive them shortly! When the students heard the news, they dropped to their knees on the concrete floor and gave thanks to the Lord for providing for them. I will never forget that moment!

When I returned home, I sought to set up a project called 'Books for Pastors' in co-operation with Africa Christian Textbooks (ACTS) to provide discounted book sets for pastors in Nigeria. Many people prayed and gave towards this project. The ministry of ACTS continues to flourish today—and I believe it is a very strategic and important one in Nigeria, with its population of around 200 million. If a pastor is strengthened and grows in leadership, he will be able to strengthen the sometimes numerous congregations that are under his care. When I think of ACTS, I think of it beginning like an acorn and developing into a strong, growing tree! In the words of William Carey, who is known as the 'father of modern missions': 'Expect great things from God. Attempt great things for God.'

Kidnap threat

The ongoing threat of kidnapping in the Niger Delta meant that I was unable to attend a pastors' conference that I had been invited to speak at or take up the opportunity of speaking on the local radio station. I was more or less confined to the compound where I lived, the church next to it, and the College just beyond that. However, the Lord used the situation for good and I was able to give myself to nurturing and discipling the eager and passionate students at WWTC which was a great delight.

One Sunday after church, a few young men were hanging around. They were not locals and it all looked unusual and very suspicious. I was expected to be at church the following Sunday—but, as I became aware of the danger involved, I was really afraid. I was very tempted to stay at home and miss church for my own safety. After reading the Word, discussing the matter with Rufus and Iris, we cried out in prayer to the Lord. The peace of God which passes all human understanding came to my mind. I was able to be present at church on Sunday, and I returned home rejoicing. All was well.

What next?

When I returned home from nearly six months in Nigeria I was physically, mentally and emotionally exhausted. I was not able to attend my home church on the Sunday because it was too much for me, so I rested at home. I couldn't really concentrate for any period of time and I felt very broken. I visited my GP who said that there was some kind of bacteria in my body. Thankfully, some three weeks later, the GP gave me the 'all clear'; I had recovered.

What was I going to do next? I had no job and no idea what I should do next. I was reading Acts 16 and noticed that a door had closed for the apostle Paul and his ministry team as they were prevented from preaching the Word in the province of Asia (verse 6). Then they tried to enter Bithynia (verse 7), but the door of opportunity closed so they arrived in Troas (verse 8). It was in Troas that the Lord spoke by means of a vision: 'Come over to Macedonia and help us' (verse 9) and an open door lay ahead for them in Macedonia (verse 10).

I knew doors were now closed for me in BCM and Mission Africa, and I was seeking guidance. Brian Smyth was now an assistant minister in Glendermott Presbyterian Church on the outskirts of Londonderry. He telephoned to tell me that there was a great need for ministers in the Presbyterian Church in Ireland, as many ministers were due to retire over the next few years. He challenged me to apply. The Lord spoke powerfully through him that an open door lay ahead in that new sphere of ministry. I decided to contact the Dean of Studies, Rev Ronnie Hetherington, to make an appointment to discuss the matter further.

On the morning of Wednesday 11 August 2010, I read Ephesians 4:1, 'I urge you to live a life worthy of the calling you have received.' Ronnie was very encouraging and I left that meeting more assured about applying to become a candidate to be a minister in the Presbyterian Church in Ireland. At the same time, I wrestled with the decision—because I didn't want to apply and be turned down. It was a huge step and the thought of failure still lingered in my mind. I needed to be sure before I applied. I remembered how King Hezekiah took the letter he had received, went up to the Temple of the Lord and spread it out before the Lord (Isaiah 37:14). Therefore, I took the application and spread it out before the Lord in prayer. I thought: I have a Bible in my hand and the Holy Spirit within me, therefore I have everything I need to be a good minister of the gospel.

I felt that it was now a step of obedience to God to move forward and that I must apply. So, in September 2010, I filled in the form and applied to become a candidate in training for the Presbyterian Church in Ireland. In many ways, I was going back to my spiritual roots. I was interviewed by the student committee from the Ballymena Presbytery, which was followed by the entrance process to Union Theological College in Belfast. Having received the news that I had been successful in my application, I was overcome and moved to tears that the Lord had opened a door for ministry within the church.

Chapter 6

FINDING LOVE

I had wanted to be married for some time, but nothing seemed to work out for me. In April 2012, I was living at home with my dad in Ahoghill. I had recently completed further studies at Belfast Bible College in Dunmurry and was now a student at Union Theological College in Belfast.

A good woman

I had gone with some friends to a restaurant near Ballymena for some dinner. Afterwards, we were making our way to our cars when a friend Roger Rossborough said to me, 'There's a good woman for you!' He pointed in the direction of Karen Anderson. I happened to have a brief conversation with Karen later that day after a Christian meeting, and again a few weeks later at friend's get-together in Bangor. Then Karen turned up at a friend's barbecue. I spent some time that evening chatting to her and I made up my mind that I should ask her out for coffee, as you do! I asked a mutual friend to ask her whether she was happy to give me her mobile number. Meanwhile, Karen, who comes from a Baptist family, had said to her mother, 'This Presbyterian minister has asked me out!' Her mother, Irene, replied, 'Well I won't be telling your father!' Karen thought about it and decided against it. The reply came back: 'no'! That was disappointing—but, as the old adage says, "A faint heart never won a fair lady"!

The next week, I bumped into Karen again and this time Karen came up to talk to me and we got on really well together. Karen sent me her mobile number the next day and we decided to arrange a date. Karen was working in Castlewellan Christian Conference centre—about forty-five miles south of Ballyclare Presbyterian Church, where I was due to begin working as a student assistant. We arranged to go for a meal in an Indian restaurant in Newcastle. After the meal, we went for a walk and then had a coffee in the Lighthouse Lounge of The Slieve Donard Hotel. The next day, I was away teaching the Bible at an Oak Hall Holiday mystery tour to the Republic of Ireland. Oak Hall is an organisation based in Otford Manor in Kent that runs Christian holidays and expeditions. For this particular holiday, there were meetings each evening and sightseeing trips during the day. I received a text from Karen that she would see me in six weeks' time. I took that to mean that she was not interested so I decided to stop texting her.

After a few days, Karen was apparently wondering why I had not texted her. She talked to our mutual friend, James Sloss, and she began texting me again. I was absolutely delighted and over the moon! We had some further dates—and, at the end of June 2012, we decided to go out together. In July, Karen was hosting a barbecue at Castlewellan Christian Conference centre for the Christian Institute and I welcomed people as well as prayed at the event. Karen and I were officially an item. A wise man said to me that evening, 'She's a keeper'!

During July and August, I regularly travelled from Ballymena to visit Karen at Castlewellan Castle. I also visited Karen's home—May's Corner just outside Rathfriland, about ten miles from Karen's work—and I spent time getting to know her parents, Irene and Graham.

On one occasion, I was talking to Graham in the dining room. Around the walls of the dining room were wedding photos of members of the family, and Graham said to me, 'I would like another one of these'.[7] I knew all was going well! In September, Karen came for the first time to a meeting in Ballyclare Presbyterian Church

7 David and Esther Anderson, Denver and Lynne Wilson, and Robin and Diane Madely.

where I was working. Karen later told me that the thought of being a minister's wife was petrifying to her. That, of course, is totally understandable.

"Will you marry me?"

In the autumn, it was evident that our relationship was blossoming and we knew that we loved each other. By April 2013, I was thinking about how I should propose to Karen. Should we go to a sandy beach where I would write in the sand, 'Will you marry me?' Should we travel to the penguin enclosure at Belfast Zoo (for I knew that Karen loves animals) where I would ask her, 'Will you marry me?' Should I take her out for a meal in a hotel and, at the end, ask her, 'Will you marry me?' I decided against all of these options!

Then I thought, Adam met Eve in the garden; that would be an ideal place! So, when Karen and I were walking in the front garden of my family home on the morning of Wednesday 3 April, I went down on one knee and asked her, 'Will you marry me?' Thankfully, she said, 'Yes!' I then proceeded to place an engagement ring on the wrong finger of the wrong hand—I was so overcome.

We came into the house and shared the news with my father, William. I then telephoned my brother, Neil, who was in South Africa with his wife, Kate, and son, James. Karen phoned her parents, Graham and Irene. We then had a celebration lunch at Leighinmohr House Hotel in Ballymena. Next, we went to see Brian Smyth and his family. Brian had recently been called to be minister of Trinity Presbyterian Church in Ahoghill. When we walked in the door, there were boxes everywhere. I am sure they thought we had come to help—but we were there on another errand! We asked Brian to conduct the wedding.

The wedding

We decided on Tuesday 23 July for our wedding day—and plans came together quickly. That was good, as we only had four months to plan everything. Karen's sister, Lynne, recommended Edenmore

Golf and Country Club as a venue. When we were shown round by the wedding co-ordinator and our hearts were soon set on this venue in its lovely countryside setting. The wedding dress was quickly chosen and we were on our way! Deciding who to include on our wedding list was a very tricky decision to make. At first, we thought about inviting just 35 guests, then it became 45 guests—but, eventually, we decided to invite over 60 guests!

The weather on the day of the wedding was sunny and warm. A Christian service was held in a room at the venue. Rev Brian Smyth conducted the ceremony and preached God's Word, Graham Anderson read the Scriptures, and Lynne and Denver Wilson sang a duet. While the photographs were taken, the guests enjoyed a golf putting competition. After the meal, David Anderson organised a family quiz. We all had lots of fun and laughter—a memorable day. I had found a real gem.[8]

We flew to Faro Airport in the Algarve in Portugal for our honeymoon. On the Saturday, we spent most of the day beside the swimming pool and, around dinner time, we walked back to our room. I noticed that my wedding ring was not on my hand. We retraced our steps and a young person even jumped into the swimming pool in search of the precious ring. A lady even said she would pray to a saint on my behalf that the ring be found! But there was no word of any ring being found. All looked lost. I had spent so long in my life waiting for a ring and now it had not even lasted a week... But all was not lost. Later, we called at the hotel reception and were told that the ring had been found in the bottom of the swimming pool!

Our first home

We returned to Northern Ireland and set up home in Newtownabbey, not far from Ballyclare Presbyterian Church where I was now a full-time assistant to the minister, Rev Robert Bell. Karen and I

8 Or, in the words of Proverbs 31:10, 'A wife of noble character who can find? She is worth far more than rubies'.

learned a lot during our time at Ballyclare and we enjoyed the ministry there. One of my first pastoral visits was to the home of Maurice and Kay Fisher. Maurice was the 'clerk of session', an elder of the church who has a close working relationship with the minister. Before I left, I read from Proverbs 3:5-6.

> *Trust in the Lord with all your heart*
> *and lean not on your own understanding;*
> *in all your way submit to him,*
> *and he will make your paths straight.*

Maurice brought out a Bible that they had been given when they were married some years earlier and the same verses, Proverbs 3:5-6, were written there. It was a reminder that the eternal God who guided Maurice and Kaye together in marriage was still guiding us in His will and still speaking to us today.

In January 2015, I became eligible to be called to a church (or churches) as a minister. What lay ahead for us?

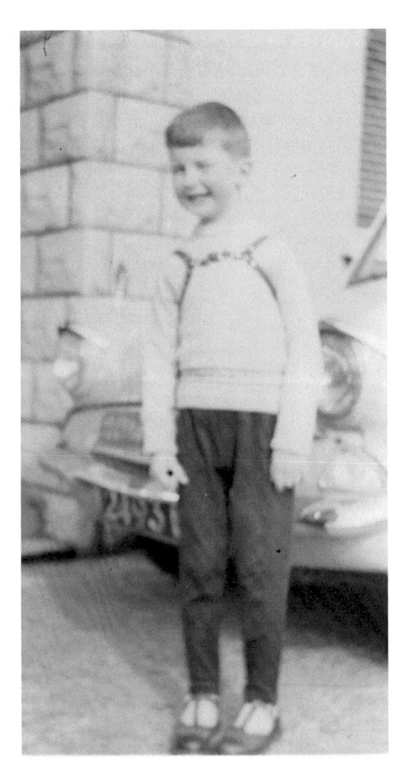

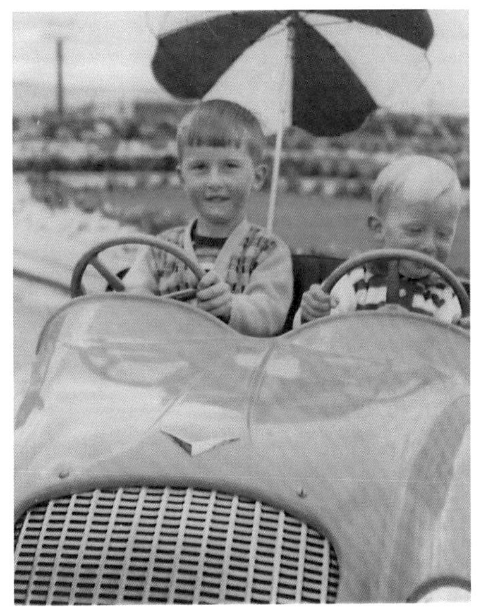

Left: It was obvious from early on that I would be tall.
Above: With my brother on holiday.
Below: My Dad, Mum and wee brother Neil.

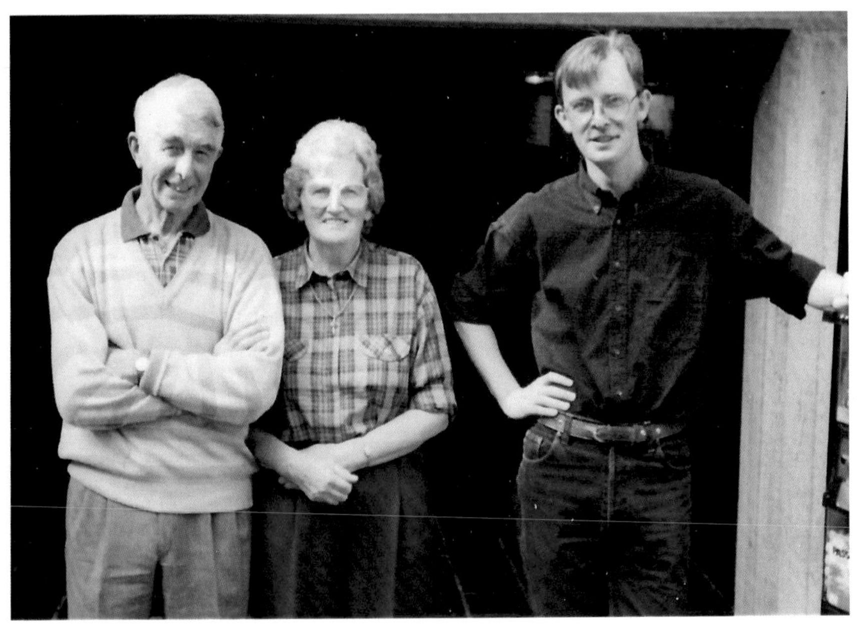

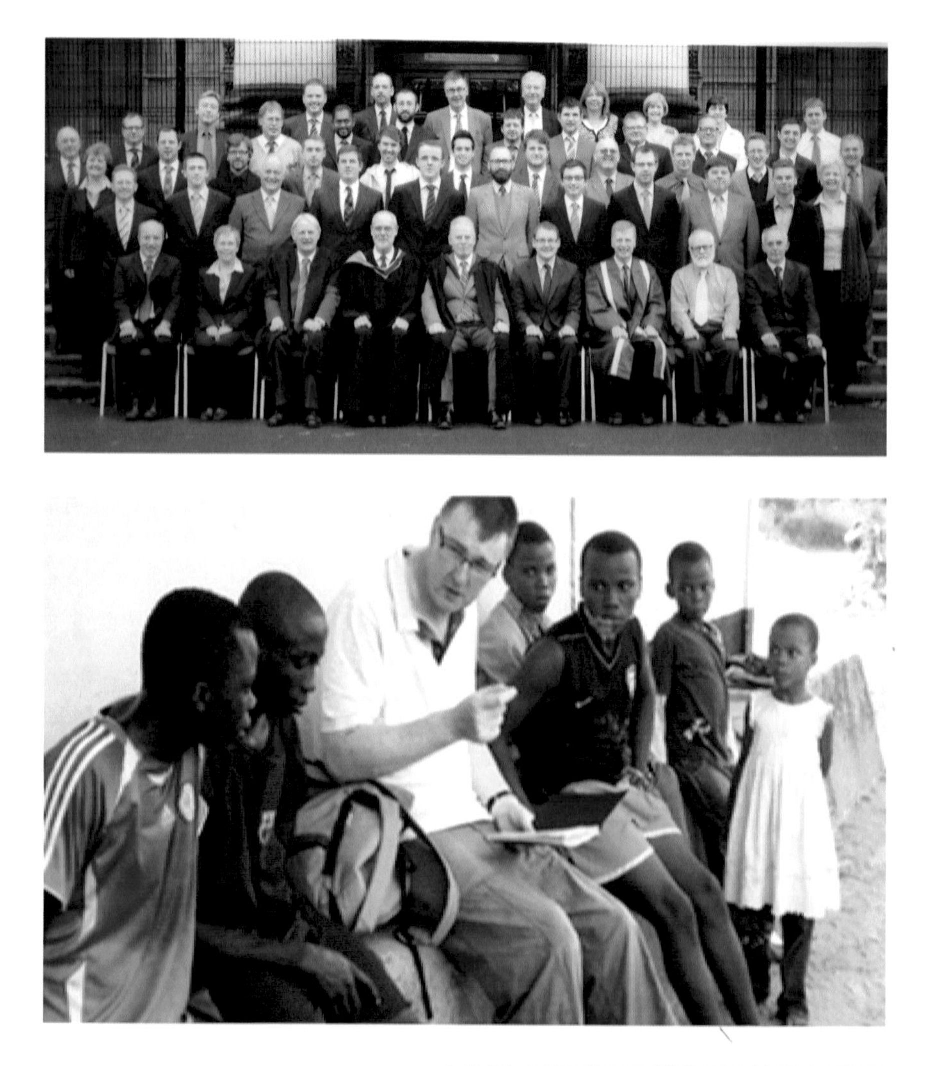

Top: Faculty and students at Union Theological College Belfast in 2012/13—the year I graduated.

Centre: Teaching the gospel to teenagers and children in Nigeria.

Right: Our family farm in the winter snow.

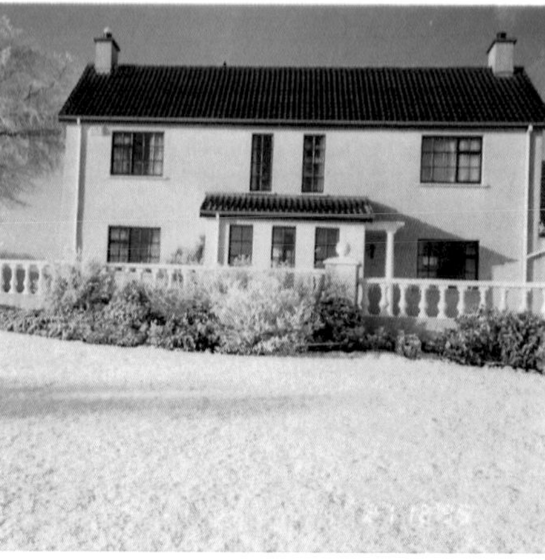

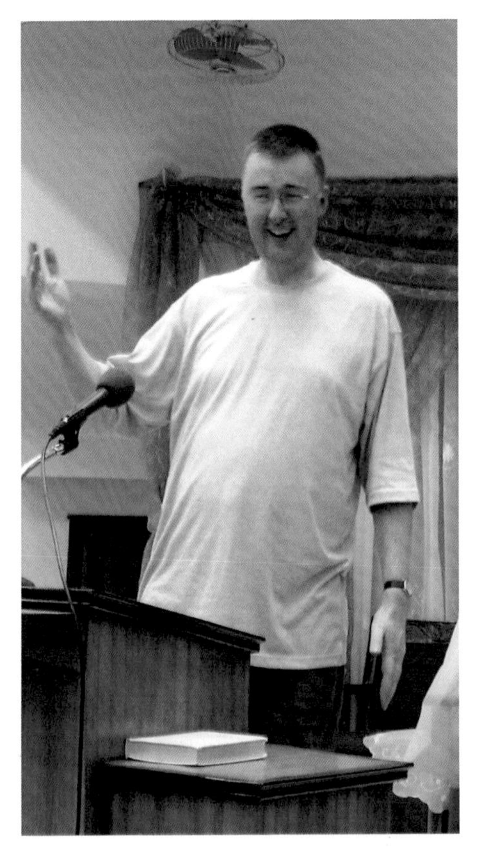

Top: Adrian standing in a Nigerian pulpit

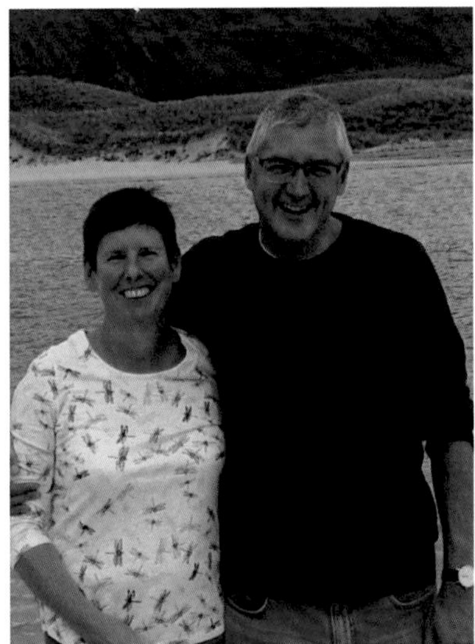

Below: My best friend Brian Smyth and his lovely wife Pamela.

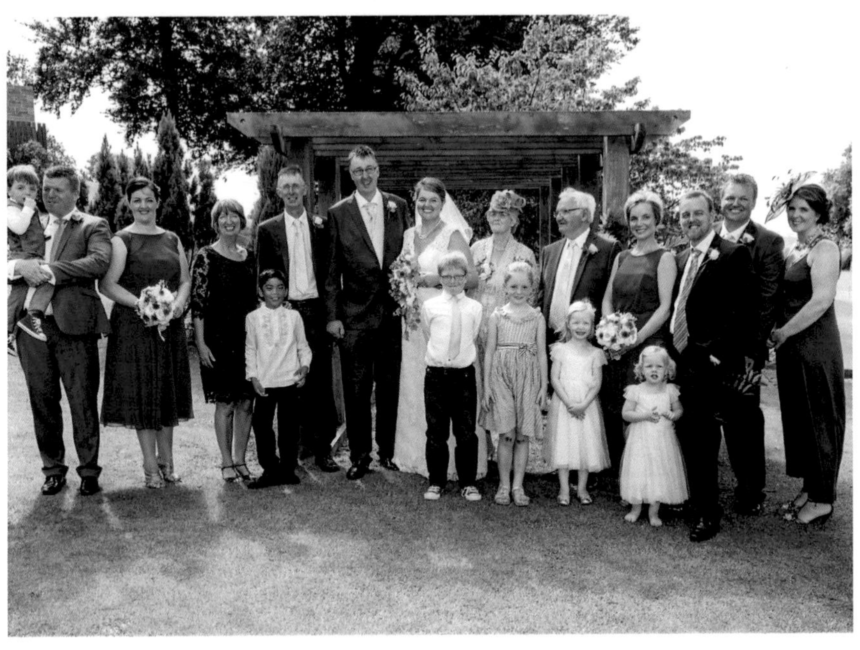

Bottom: The Adger and Anderson families celebrating the happy day.

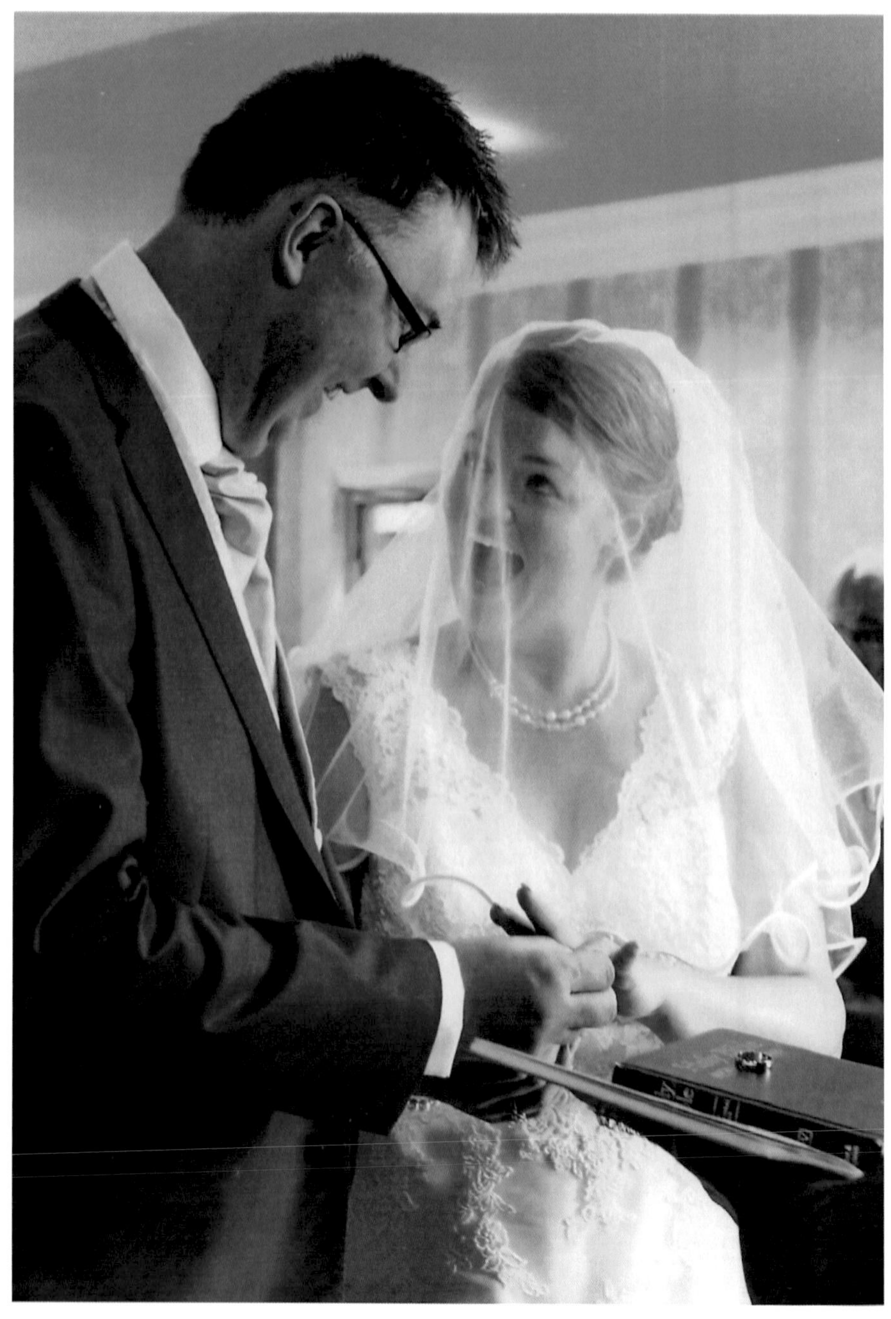

With Karen on our wedding day: the ring fits!

Chapter 7

Finding our home

I was confused and unsure where the Lord would have me to serve. I called in to see Irene and Graham Anderson, Karen's parents, who have been a tremendous support to us both, along with the rest of the family. I asked Graham, with whom I have a very close friendship, for some advice regarding guidance.

He told me about when his old pastor, Willie Mullan, was living in east Belfast and had been reading about the apostle Peter in Acts 10: 'three men seek thee. Arise therefore, and get thee down, and go with them, doubting nothing: for I have sent them' (Acts 10:19-20, KJV).

Very soon after, three men from Lurgan Baptist Church came to the door of Willie's home and called him to be their pastor! This inspired me—so, on 11 February 2015, I prayed to the Lord: 'Send three men to come and ask me to be their minister.' As I read Acts 10, verse 32 also stood out for me: 'Simon the tanner lives by the sea.' I wondered, would the church be by the sea?

On the way to the land of mountains

Following one interview that led nowhere, a visit from a delegation from two churches in County Tyrone and various conversations, I was offered an interview with the elders of Clough and Seaforde churches, County Down, on Friday 20 March 2015. Nine other candidates were also called for interview. From my perspective, my interview was the worst I had given in my life! I felt I hadn't said all that I had intended to say and that I had given them an incomplete picture. Yet, to my surprise, the elders asked me to speak at the two churches. A sovereign Lord was at work guiding His servant.

Two other candidates were also asked to speak and conduct morning and evening services on separate Sundays. Having listened to all three candidates, the church would hold a congregational meeting of church members and prayerfully choose who they should call to be their new minister. When I conducted Sunday worship services at these churches at the end of April, I really enjoyed being there and being with the people. The next day, the members of Clough and Seaforde churches gathered to choose their minister. That morning, Karen shared with me her devotions from Deuteronomy 11.

> [8] *Observe therefore all the commands I am giving you today, so that you may have the strength to go in and take over the land that you are crossing the Jordan to possess,* [9] *and so that you may live long in the land the Lord swore to your ancestors to give to them and their descendants, a land flowing with milk and honey.* [10] *The land you are entering to take over is not like the land of Egypt, from which you have come, where you planted your seed and irrigated it by foot as in a vegetable garden.* [11] *But the land you are crossing the Jordan to take possession of is a land of mountains and valleys that drinks rain from heaven.* [12] *It is a land the Lord your God cares for; the eyes of the Lord your God are continually on it from the beginning of the year to its end.* (Deuteronomy 11:8-12)

I particularly noticed the word 'today' in verse 8. And, in verse 11, 'the land you are crossing ... to take is a land of mountains'—the 'land of mountains'... When Karen and I read that, we worshipped God for we were sure the Lord was leading us to a land of mountains that day—the Slieve Donard mountain range dominates the skyline when you are at these two churches.

That evening, the church members voted to 'issue a unanimous call' for me to be their minister. The convenor of the churches, Rev James Hyndman, telephoned me soon after to tell me the news. I immediately said, 'Yes!' As I was an assistant minister in Ballyclare Presbyterian (which is in the Carrickfergus Presbytery) at the time, the call was presented at the Carrickfergus Presbytery meeting just over a week later. It was supported by three men—three elders in Clough and Seaforde churches. It was accepted by me as I knew God had sent them, fulfilling God's Word to me in Acts 10. In mid-June 2015, I was ordained and installed as minister of Clough and Seaforde Presbyterian churches by a commission from the Down Presbytery. My family, including my father and brother, were present for the service. I had become especially close to my father, having gone home to live with him in Ahoghill following my mother's death in 2004, until my marriage to Karen.

A courageous end

In March 2016, I learned that my father was diagnosed with asbestosis, a form of cancer. He had worked most of his life in the construction industry and had handled asbestos. There was no understanding of health and safety issues then and, at some stage, asbestos fibres had been breathed in and brought about this condition years later. When I heard the news, I was shocked. I could not speak and was in tears. I felt very down. Having shed many tears, I started to feel a little better. I was trying to come to terms with the news.

My father faced his cancer with courage. For some months, he was unable to attend church. On a number of occasions, he came and stayed with us for short periods. He always loved being home. Incredibly, in October and early November, he was driving and out at church for the harvest celebrations and enjoyed attending the Lisnafillon Mission Hall for their evening service. He received amazing support from friends and neighbours. However, at the beginning of December, he had a fall in his home. He was admitted into Antrim Area Hospital. A few days later, when I was visiting him in the hospital, I read Psalm 121.

I lift my eyes to the mountains—
where does my help come from?
My help comes from the Lord,
the maker of heaven and earth. (Psalm 121:1-2)

William prayed to the Lord his Maker and Saviour and gave thanks for His care of him over the years, and he prayed for God's mercy to be shown to his family. Neil had flown from Exeter and spent time with him over the weekend. On Monday, when Karen and I visited him again, he said to us, 'I'll recover.' We left him just after 8.30 pm and were travelling home by car when Karen received the news from the hospital that William had passed away at 9.15 pm. Later that evening, when we shared the news, Karen's mother Irene said, 'He has recovered all right.' He was now at home with the Lord.

As a husband, father, grandfather and elder in the church, my father had served the Lord well. He is now absent from the body and present with the Lord (2 Corinthians 5:8). Rev Brian Smyth spoke powerfully on 2 Timothy 4 at the service of thanksgiving in Trinity Presbyterian Church.

I have fought the good fight, I have finished the race, I have kept the faith. Now there is in store for me the crown of righteousness. (2 Timothy 4:7-8)

I am thankful for the great support I received from family, friends and our precious church family as I grieved the loss. I felt the cruelness of death taking my father whom I loved and who showed me incredible support. I longed to talk to him again—the finality of death is hard to come to terms with. We grieve—yet we grieve with hope of a new heaven and a new earth, where God's people dwell for evermore:

Then I saw 'a new heaven and a new earth,' for the first heaven and the first earth had passed away, and there was no longer any sea. I saw the Holy City, the new Jerusalem, coming down out of heaven from God, prepared as a bride

> *beautifully dressed for her husband. And I heard a loud voice from the throne saying, 'Look! God's dwelling place is now among the people, and he will dwell with them. They will be his people, and God himself will be with them and be their God. "He will wipe every tear from their eyes. There will be no more death" or mourning or crying or pain, for the old order of things has passed away'.*
>
> (*Revelation 21:1-4*)

One day there will be a great reunion when God's people will be together with their Lord and Saviour. Serving the Lord in Clough and Seaforde Presbyterian churches is a joy and privilege. The two clerks of Session, David Croskery and William McCall, have been a tremendous support to us along with the other elders and people in the churches.[9]

Where is my home?

As I face incurable and inoperable cancer at this time, a question I have been thinking about is: where is home? Where is my home? During my early years, I lived with mum and dad and my brother Neil in a bungalow on my grandparents' farm outside Ballymena. Then we moved into the farmhouse and, for many years, that was the family home—the place where I belonged, the place of special memories, the place of love and laughter, the place where I felt most comfortable and relaxed. When I walked through the door, I knew I was home.

However, a lot has changed over the years. My brother moved to Scotland when he was eighteen years old and is now a professor at Exeter University. My mum died on Christmas Day 2004 and my father died on 12 December 2016. When I go back to that building now, I don't find a home. It's just a building. It's a cold and empty house. Yes, the bricks and the mortar and the walls and the tiled

9 I thank God for all the elders, who also include: Bruce Mitchell, Tony Watson, Geoffrey Brown, Les Drew, Brian Dumigan, Stephen Heenan, Francis Johnston, Rodney Martin, John McKibben and, elder emeritus, Dr Ronnie Hamilton.

roof are there—but it's a house, not a home. I don't really belong there anymore. My heart isn't there. I will always have cherished memories—but it's not my home.

Then when I married Karen, we moved to live in Newtownabbey. It was our first home together and we have happy memories of living in Ashford Lodge. However, today someone else is living in the house. It's a building—and it's no longer our home.

Since 2015, we have been living in the church manse, just outside Clough, on the Drumcaw Road—and we both loving living here. There is a field in the front with sheep in it and, at the side, a field with cattle in it. We are at home here in the countryside. This is a very special place for us where special memories are being made. This is where I feel most comfortable and happy. It is a place we love, it is a place where we belong. Yet, is this really my 'home'?

In the book of Genesis 12, we read about a man called Abraham who lived in a tent. Now a tent has no foundations, it is a temporary structure—and Abraham moved from place to place. He had no permanent address, no postcode. He simply believed in the Lord and he was looking forward to the city whose architect and builder is God (Hebrews 11:10).

In Psalm 23:6, David writes about 'dwelling in the house of the Lord forever'. Whose house is David speaking about? It is the house of the Lord, the house that belongs to God. It is the abode of God—and David is speaking about living there forever, never leaving that house.

Then in John's gospel, we read about how the Lord Jesus Christ said to his disciples:

> *My Father's house has many rooms; if that were not so, would I have told you that I am going there to prepare a place for you?* (*John 14:2*)

So now Jesus is speaking about His Father's house, the place where God lives and dwells in heaven, God's eternal home. This is a real place—a permanent place, a prepared place for a prepared people.

A permanent home

And so I realise that all the places that I've lived in the world are only temporary. It is God's home that is permanent and eternal. One day soon, I will go to my eternal home in heaven. That is where I really belong. As the old song goes:

This world is not my home I'm just a passing through
My treasures are laid up somewhere beyond the blue.[10]

But the question that I have is this: why am I so confident that heaven is my home? Can I be really sure of going to heaven—or not? It is God's Word that assures me that everyone who trusts in the Lord is going to heaven. What do I mean by 'trusts in the Lord'? I mean everyone who has renounced their sin, turned away from their wrongdoing, received Jesus Christ as their Saviour and Lord, and believes that Jesus died on the cross of Calvary for their sins and rose again from the dead on the third day.

I want to ask you a searching question: are you sure of going to heaven? Are you prepared? Jesus also warned that those who are unprepared to meet God face eternity in an awful place called hell, where they suffer the wrath of God because of their sin (Luke 16:19-31).

One morning, I looked out of the window of my family home and there was mist everywhere. I couldn't see anything. I couldn't see the main road in front of the house, I couldn't see the garden—because of the white mist. In the afternoon, the mist disappeared, and the road and garden were clearly visible. James 4:14 reminds us that our life is like that mist. We are only here on earth a little while, just a very short time. And even the longest life lived in this world is incredibly short, compared with eternity. So now is the time to prepare to meet God. Don't delay.

10 Jim Reeves, 'This World Is Not My Home'.

Chapter 8

Finding hope and joy in the midst of cancer

After I received a diagnosis of incurable cancer, my mind was full of questions. Will I ever know joy again in my life? Will I have to carry this heavy burden with me for the rest of my time on earth? Why me? Is God punishing me? Am I finished? Should I pray for healing or not? What shall I pray? With the minister unwell, will our church perhaps dwindle and decline? Where does my confidence really lie? So many questions... Here are a few reflections on some of the questions I've been considering since my diagnosis.

Will I ever know joy again in my life?

One of my initial thoughts was this: will I ever know joy again in my life? Will I now have to carry this heavy burden with me always? I was filled with sadness, grief and a sense of loss. I also knew that this burden was too heavy for us to carry on our own. At first, we shared the news with family and my best friend, Rev Brian Smyth. Then, on Sunday evening, at the joint evening service in Clough Presbyterian church hall, we had a time of praise and I shared briefly from Psalm 13. After that, I shared with the church family and we had a time of 'open prayer' where anyone in the church family could pray as they felt led. I was in tears and so were others in the church. Margaret McCombe, a former missionary in Nepal, read from Isaiah 43. Verse 2 stood out:

When you pass through the waters,
I will be with you;
and when you pass through the rivers,
they will not sweep over you.
When you walk through the fire
you will not be burned;
the flames will not set you ablaze.

I stopped crying and felt a peace and joy come over me. I closed the service in prayer and we sang a hymn. Karen and I are not alone The Lord is definitely with us. Yes, there would be more tears and struggles—yet we knew the very presence of the Lord. We were beginning to turn a corner and come to terms with the news. We had been totally disorientated but we were beginning to find our equilibrium again. It is a very hard road that we are on, yet the support of our precious church family and so many others is amazing.

The church family has been carrying our burden (Galatians 6:2) and they have been showing us such love. The elders called the two churches to fast and pray on a Thursday in November 2017. The elders then came to the manse, they prayed over me and anointed me with oil according to James 5:14-15. There was a powerful sense of the presence and power of God in the room. The Lord has sustained us every step of the way. In all this, I have known joy again—and the Lord has provided a precious church family to help carry our burden.

Cast your cares on the Lord and he will sustain you.
(Psalm 55:22)

Why me?

What had I done wrong? Why now? I had only been married a short time and I love my wife deeply. I had only become a minister a short time before and, by God's grace, the churches were going so well. I felt as if I was being cut down in the midst of life. I felt as if I was being robbed of so much. I felt it was so unfair. Yet, as I reflect on this, I realise that I don't have all the answers to my questions—but neither do I have to. God Himself is enough. As I belong to the Lord, I have everything I need (Psalm 23:1).

Christ is enough for me,
Everything I need is in you,
Everything I need.[11]

These are lines from a song sung by Proclaim youth choir in my home church one Sunday. Even when I don't understand, I am able to worship—for I have been set free.

Even when I don't understand it all and my faith wavers, I have my loving Father in heaven whom I am able to trust completely, knowing without a shadow of a doubt that He is working out everything for the good of His people. Not everything that happens to us feels good—far from it—but God is at work in all our circumstances to accomplish His good purpose. That 'good' is to mould and shape our character more and more into the image of God's dear Son, the Lord Jesus Christ, and also bring us to final glory. *Hallelujah.*

> *And we know that in all things God works for the good of those who love him, who have been called according to his purpose. For those God foreknew he also predestined to be conformed to the image of his Son, that he might be the firstborn among many brothers and sisters. And those he predestined, he also called; those he called, he also justified; those he justified, he also glorified.* (Romans 8:28-30)

There are times when I feel that I am being robbed of the years ahead and robbed of so much in life, that I am missing out and losing out compared with other people. Yet, when I do that, I am failing to fully understand and appreciate the incredible benefits and privileges that I have. I have found a pearl of great value: the Lord Jesus Christ (Matthew 13:45, 46). I have received a new iden-

11 Reuben Morgan and Jonas Myrin, 'Christ is Enough', Hillsong Music Publishing, 2012.

tity as a child of the King, and a new family of brothers and sisters in the Lord. I have gained eternal life—something that I am so unworthy of. I will definitely not miss out in eternity and final glory. And that is what really matters.

> *When we've been there ten thousand years,*
> *Bright shining as the sun,*
> *We've no less days to sing God's praise*
> *Than when we first begun.*[12]

Is God punishing me?

At first, I thought that I must have done wrong and that God must be punishing me for some sin that I had committed. Then I thought back to the weekend before. There had been a Child Evangelism Conference at Rathfriland Baptist Church, County Down—Karen's home church—and I spoke at the meeting. I had not been sure what passage to choose and had wrestled with what I should share from God's Word. I finally decided on Exodus 17:8-16 which is about the defeat of the Amalekites by Moses and the importance of prayer. David Crutchley (the local Child Evangelism Fellowship worker) and others had encouraged me afterwards.[13]

I realised that if God had chosen to use me one minute, then He hadn't disowned me the next. He promised to never leave me (Hebrews 13:5). In any case, Jesus Christ had already taken the punishment and penalty that all my sins deserved on the cross at Calvary. Jesus had already died in my place—so God could not punish me again, as His wrath has already been satisfied at the cross. It wasn't God punishing me at all—for he loves me with unconditional love.

Am I finished?

As the days passed, I wondered whether I would ever be useful again.

---

12 John Newton, 'Amazing Grace', 1779.

13 David and Olivia Crutchley are local directors for Child Evangelism Fellowship Ireland in the Mourne area and have been an encouragement to me.

Am I finished? Will the Lord ever use me in His service again? Is it all over? On Boxing Day 2017, I was talking to two men (not from our congregations) who said that they heard that this would be my last sermon and that I was resigning as a minister in the church at the end of December. I said that was not the case. But I wondered, had the Lord finished with me? The next day, I was going to the City Hospital for a scan and what did I find myself reading in the Scriptures..? My reading was from John 21:

> [15] *Jesus said to Simon Peter, 'Simon son of John, do you love me more than these?'*
> *'Yes, Lord,' he said, 'you know that I love you.'*
> *Jesus said, 'Feed my lambs.'*
> [16] *Again Jesus said, 'Simon son of John, do you love me?'*
> *He answered, 'Yes, Lord, you know that I love you.'*
> *Jesus said, 'Take care of my sheep.'*
> [17] *The third time he said to him, 'Simon son of John, do you love me?'*
> *Peter was hurt because Jesus asked him the third time, 'Do you love me?' He said, 'Lord, you know all things; you know that I love you.'*
> *Jesus said, 'Feed my sheep.'*

'Feed my lambs' (verse 15), 'Take care of my sheep' (verse 16), 'Feed my sheep' (verse 17). These words for this servant of the Lord seemed bizarre and impossible for me to do in the light of my diagnosis and the fact that I was beginning my chemotherapy in January 2018. Yet I knew they were very relevant. I was now sure God was renewing His call upon my life and calling me to serve Him afresh by providing the spiritual food of God's Word for his flock.

The opportunities I have had to share God's Word and be a witness for Christ have been incredible. When the consultant gave me the news of incurable cancer, I was honestly able to say, 'I am not afraid of dying because I know where I am going. I know I am going to heaven—not because I am a minister, but because, at the age of twenty-two, I gave my life to Jesus Christ.' I have had the opportunity to share my faith in Jesus Christ with many in the medical profession.

In 2018, a friend said to me that I had a story to tell and I should put it on social media. I didn't believe him or think it was a good idea. He kept on saying it—and I began to think that perhaps he had a point. The elders agreed and supported the project. I was led to Jonny Sanlon, a videographer, who has helped me to put my story into a series of five short videos which have been released on our church website, our Facebook page, on Vimeo and on YouTube. The response has been unbelievable. One video called 'Finding Hope' has had over 15,000 views. The videos have been viewed in Argentina, Canada, United States of America, Mexico, Australia, Thailand, Nigeria, Kenya, Russia, Finland, Italy, Estonia, etc. One day, my work for God on earth will be finished, but until then I will serve my Lord and Saviour, Jesus Christ.

Should I pray for healing or not? What shall I pray?

One big question we have wrestled with is the question of healing. Should I pray for healing or not? What should I pray? I reflected on this issue in the April 2019 edition of the *Presbyterian Herald* magazine. Karen and I both felt that we should pray for healing.

> *I don't feel that as Christians we should be fatalistic and just accept things. God is interested in us physically, emotionally, mentally and spiritually, so there's a wholeness to us. James 5 says, 'Is anyone among you sick? Let them call the elders of the church to pray over them…' I think we have to be led by the Holy Spirit as well though. And it's not just about asking 'heal me', it's about praising God and rejoicing in what Jesus Christ has done for us. We also rejoice that God is Sovereign and we want to delight in doing His will.*[14]

Whatever God's will is… That is of paramount importance, because

14 Sarah Harding, 'Joy in the Trial', Presbyterian Herald, April 2019. Quoted with permission.

we know that God has plans to use us both when we are sick and when we are well. Then, one day, we will be with Jesus Christ which is 'better by far', when we will know ultimate healing and have a perfect glorified body (Philippians 1:23, 1 Corinthians 15:51-57). Each day that the Lord gives is a gift from God, and we should pray that we might glorify God and enjoy our relationship with Him in our lives. We acknowledge that we sin in thought, word and deed and that we need the Lord's forgiveness. We should pray that we might grow in holiness and that God might use us in His service.

Two mnemonics that I have found helpful are these—PRAY and ACTS:

P*raise the Lord*
R*epent of sin*
A*sk for others*
Y*ourself*

A*doration of God*
C*onfess sin*
T*hanksgiving for what the Lord has done*
S*upplication (praying for others)*

With the minister unwell, perhaps the church will dwindle and be on the decline?

My next question was this: is the church waning? Not so, it seems. God's work in His church is not all about us! During 2018, I was receiving chemotherapy treatment and I found mornings difficult as I was fatigued. Yet on Sunday morning, I was buoyed up by the prayers of God's people and was strengthened by the Lord to keep on preaching.

In 2018, we started our 'home groups'—weekly meetings in the homes of church members to study God's Word and pray, for spiritual encouragement and friendship. They were encouraging times. Two new elders (Geoffrey Brown and Les Drew) were ordained in Clough. An American team from Pittsburgh USA and Kentucky Christian University came to the church and served with us, while they stayed at Murlough House in Dundrum. The Church Facebook page has grown and now has over 700 followers.

My illness has resulted in greater unity among the church families in Clough and Seaforde, and our faith in Christ has deepened by God's grace. I now co-ordinate the pastoral care in the church. I am so thankful for the amazing team of elders (led by David Croskery in Seaforde and by William McCall in Clough) who have carried out additional pastoral responsibilities, especially in visiting the sick. I was in hospital twice during 2018 with infections—but I am so thankful that the Lord has sustained me.

New people have come to the churches, reminding me that the battle is the Lord's and the church belongs to Christ who promises to build His church and that nothing will thwart His plans and purposes (Matthew 16:18). The church is so precious to the Lord (Acts 20:28).

Where does my confidence really lie?

Having received the difficult scan result in early January 2019, the week drew on and I started to think about what Bible passage I should share with my brothers and sisters at church that Sunday. What should I say? I felt led to the passage Philippians 1:1-11 which the new home groups had been studying that Wednesday evening. One particular verse (verse 6) stood out for me:

Being confident of this that he who began a good work in you will carry it on to completion until the day of Christ Jesus.

And I asked myself, 'Where does my confidence for the future lie?' Did it lie in the medical team caring for me? I am so thankful for the dedication and commitment to the medical team at the Cancer Centre at the Belfast City Hospital—but that wasn't the source of my confidence.

Did my confidence lie in the new immunotherapy treatment I was starting? I am so thankful for the specialists who are bringing out new drugs in the fight against cancer—but, no, my confidence wasn't in the new medication either.

Did it lie in the strength of my faith? No, it didn't because, at times, my faith does falter and is weak. God's Word reminded me that my confidence is in another. It is in Jesus Christ. My confidence lay in the fact that He who began a good work in me, and saved me by his grace, will carry it on until I see Him face to face.

My confidence is in the fact that He is working out His plans and purposes in my life and He will carry it on to completion. No cancer can thwart the plans or purposes of God for my life—in fact, it is part of those plans which will bring me to final glory when I will see the Lord Jesus Christ face to face and worship Him who is altogether lovely.

I felt great peace and joy as I considered this wonderful text. I felt lifted up and buoyed by the support and prayers of God's people.

When Satan tempts me to despair
and tells me of the guilt within,
Upward I look and see Him there
who made an end to all my sin.
Because the sinless Saviour died
my sinful soul is counted free,
For God, the just, is satisfied
to look on Him and pardon me.[15]

When Satan tempts me to despair and whispers in my ear, 'You are worthless, you are valueless, you are a failure, you are useless, you are no good, you are helpless, you are hopeless, you are finished', when he tells me of the guilt within me, what do I do? 'Upward I look'—and I see Jesus Christ, who dealt with all my sin. And because of that, I am still able to rejoice and will always rejoice. I have this assurance: the best is yet to come for all the people of God; for all whose faith is in the glorious name of Jesus Christ. My

15 'Before The Throne of God Above', original words by Charitie Lees Bancroft (1841-92), alternate words and music by Vikki Cook ©1997 Sovereign Grace Worship.

name doesn't matter. My name doesn't count. But the name of Jesus. There's no greater name. Let us all place our hope and confidence in a glorious Saviour and Lord.

Appendix

Finding encouragement in difficult times

Bible passages

Here are some of the Bible passages that I have found helpful in these past months and over the years. I hope they will bring the Lord's comfort to you.

The day after my bleak diagnosis, Karen and I read these words in **Ephesians 3:20-21** and they reminded us that the Lord was still at work in our lives and that He had not finished with us. These verses encouraged us to not give up praying:

> *Now to him who is able to do immeasurably more than all we ask or imagine, according to his power that is at work within us, to him be glory in the church and in Christ Jesus throughout all generations, for ever and ever! Amen.*

The Lord used these words in **Isaiah 43:1-2** to lift me up when I was down:

> *But now, this is what the Lord says—*
> *he who created you, Jacob,*
> *he who formed you, Israel:*
> *'Do not fear, for I have redeemed you;*
> *I have summoned you by name; you are mine.*
> *When you pass through the waters,*
> *I will be with you*

and when you pass through the rivers,
they will not sweep over you.
When you walk through the fire,
you will not be burned;
the flames will not set you ablaze.'

An elder went out of his way to come to our home to share these words in **Psalm 41:3** which I have reflected on and found encouragement in during the times that I was low in spirit:

The Lord sustains them on their sick-bed
and restores them from their bed of illness.

In August 2018, I felt so tired and weary that I was contemplating giving up the ministry I am involved in—but then I read these words in **Titus 1:2-3**, which spurred me on:

The hope of eternal life ... which now at his appointed season he has brought to light through the preaching entrusted to me by the command of God our Saviour.

In a time of confusion and perplexity regarding the future, the Lord used these words in **Acts 16:9-10** to guide me to an open door of opportunity:

During the night Paul had a vision of a man of Macedonia standing and begging him, 'Come over to Macedonia and help us.' After Paul had seen the vision, we got ready at once to leave for Macedonia, concluding that God had called us to preach the gospel to them.

In times of anxiety over the years the Lord has strengthened me through these verses in **Philippians 4:4-7**:

Rejoice in the Lord always. I will say it again: Rejoice! Let your gentleness be evident to all. The Lord is near. Do not be anxious about anything, but in every situation, by prayer and petition, with thanksgiving, present your requests to

> *God. And the peace of God, which transcends all understanding, will guard your hearts and your minds in Christ Jesus.*

During my time of grief after the death of my mum in 2004, the Lord comforted me through this verse (**Psalm 34:18**):

> *The Lord is close to the broken-hearted and saves those who are crushed in spirit.*

One evening, I struggled to sleep as I thought I had let many people down and I felt guilty for my action. After I confessed my sin, I found great peace as I relied upon this verse (**1 John 1:7**):

> *But if we walk in the light, as he is in the light, we have fellowship with one another, and the blood of Jesus, his Son, purifies us from all sin.*

There have been many been times that I have felt inadequate and uncertain. For example, before leaving my career in accountancy to serve the Lord in a new way, before travelling to Nigeria to speak, and before a number of important interviews in the church, these verses in **Exodus 4:10-12** have encouraged me to step forward.

> *Moses said to the Lord, 'Pardon your servant, Lord. I have never been eloquent, neither in the past nor since you have spoken to your servant. I am slow of speech and tongue.' The Lord said to him, 'Who gave human beings their mouths? Who makes them deaf or mute? Who gives them sight or makes them blind? Is it not I, the Lord? Now go; I will help you speak and will teach you what to say.'*

Before submitting the application form to be a candidate in training for the Presbyterian Church in Ireland, I needed direction. I read about Hezekiah in **Isaiah 37:14-15**—and I took my application form, laid it on the kitchen table and prayed. The Lord gave me peace and led me the right way.

> *Hezekiah received the letter from the messengers and read it. Then he went up to the temple of the Lord and spread it out before the Lord. And Hezekiah prayed to the Lord.*

There are times when I have felt timid, afraid and lacked confidence. The Lord has used this verse to reassure me (**2 Timothy 1:7**):

> *For the Spirit God gave us does not make us timid, but gives us power, love and self-discipline.*

At the beginning of January 2007, the Lord revealed to me that He had new things for me in the future. I had no idea what those plans were. A short-term mission trip to Nigeria would lie ahead to begin with! Maybe the Lord also wants to do new things in your life. **Isaiah 43:18-19** says this:

> *Forget the former things;*
> *do not dwell on the past.*
> *See, I am doing a new thing!*
> *Now it springs up; do you not perceive it?*
> *I am making a way in the wilderness*
> *and streams in the wasteland.*

Prayers

Some people like written prayers. Here is a prayer of commitment:

> *I admit that I am a sinner who deserves to be forsaken by a holy and righteous God—and that I deserve hell itself because of my sin. I now turn away from my sin in hatred of it. I believe that the Lord Jesus Christ died on the cross of Calvary in my place and took the punishment my sins deserve. He bore the wrath of God in my place and then rose from the dead on the third day. Thank you, Jesus, for your amazing love for me. Now I ask you to be my Saviour and Lord of my life for ever. Amen*

And a prayer for courage:

Heavenly Father, I confess that I lack courage to face this extreme difficulty, so I ask for grace to help in my time of need. I thank you that you are the Sovereign God who is in control and who is working out your purposes in the world and in my life. I praise you for your love for me, as I am so unworthy of your great salvation found in Jesus Christ. Grant me courage, strength and wisdom in order to please you and to delight in doing your will in my life. Empower me by your Holy Spirit that my life will bear witness to my family, friends and neighbours—so that those walking in Christ will be encouraged, and those walking in darkness will be drawn to the truth. Amen

Videos

A friend, Jonny Sanlon, has helped me to put my story into a series of short videos. A number of people have told me that they have found these to be very helpful. You can watch them at any of the following links:

- our church website (https://www.cloughandseaforde.com/finding-series)
- our church Facebook page (https://www.facebook.com/CloughandSeafordePresbyterian)
- Jonny Sanlon's Vimeo channel (https://vimeo.com/album/5728594)
- YouTube: (https://www.youtube.com and search for 'Adrian Adger Clough and Seaforde')

Acknowledgements and thanks

Karen and I want to our express our heartfelt appreciation to those who have prayed, encouraged and supported us from a wide spectrum of evangelical churches.

I am so thankful to Rev Dr Sid Garland for guiding me along this process of producing a book. He has been a tremendous mentor to me and has given me great advice to enable this book to be written and printed.

I want to express my deep gratitude to Mary Davis for the godly way she has helped in producing this manuscript. Mary's tremendous skill, expertise and assistance was invaluable in bringing this manuscript to completion. I greatly appreciate Tim Thornborough for his wisdom in guiding me through the process from the completion of the manuscript to the printing of the book.

I want to thank videographer Jonny Sanlon for his help in the production of the photographs for the book.

Words cannot express my great appreciation of my wife, Karen, who has been amazing every step of the way and has been such a supportive as well as encouraging wife to me. She has been patient in listening to me as I have read a portion of the manuscript to her. Karen's advice has been indispensable as we have discussed and weighed up the best words to use.

Copies of this book are available from:

All **Faith Mission** bookshops in Northern Ireland
www.faithmission.org

Belfast City Mission
5th Floor, Glengall Exchange, 3 Glengall Street,
Belfast BT12 5AB
Tel 028 9032 0557

Covenanter Bookshop
Covenanterbooks.com
37 Knockbracken Road,
Carryduff, Belfast BT8 6SE
Tel 028 9081 4110

Evangelical Bookshop
15 College Square East,
Belfast BT1 6DD
Tel 028 9032 0529

ICM Books
www.icmbooksdirect.co.uk

Mission Africa
14 Glencregagh Court,
Belfast BT6 OPA
Tel 028 9040 2850

Ards Evangelical Bookshop
48 Frances Street,
Newtownards BT23 7DN
Tel 028 9181 7530

Beulah Bookshop
25 Central Promenade,
Newcastle, BT33 0AA
Tel 028 4372 2629

The Secret Place
18 Rashee Road,
Ballyclare BT39 9HJ
Tel 028 9335 2170